Praise for Z...

"Enchanting—that is the only way to describe the eight-year-old twins at the heart of Gail McCormick's memoir. When they creep off the plane that has flown them from the Chernobyl fallout zone to Seattle for a summer of fresh air, Gail's life changes forever. The book is also a true story of love and loss and restoration. There are ups and downs, joy and sorrows. The author handles them all with a deft touch that illuminates and inspires hope."
—ELLEN BARKER, author of *East of Troost: A Novel* and *Still Needs Work: A Novel*

"Giving birth is not the only way to become a mother, as Gail McCormick proves in this engaging memoir. This is a beautifully written memoir about an important subject, especially in these days of war between Ukraine and Russia. While shining a light on truths that cannot be spoken where Vika and Maria live, McCormick also offers an encouraging Plan B for couples who struggle with infertility."
—SUE FAGALDE LICK, author of *Childless by Marriage* and *No Way Out of This: Loving a Partner with Alzheimer's*

"Gail McCormick's memoir reminds any woman who has yearned for children of her own that there are many ways to 'mother.' When one dream ends, an extraordinary life may begin."
—MELANIE NOTKIN, author of *Otherhood: Modern Women Finding a New Kind of Happiness*

Zoya's
Gift

Zoya's Gift

A MEMOIR

Building a Bridge to a Global Family

GAIL McCORMICK

SHE WRITES PRESS

Published 2024
Printed in the United States of America
Print ISBN: 978-1-64742-682-8
E-ISBN: 978-1-64742-683-5
Library of Congress Control Number: 2023919039

For information, address:
She Writes Press
1569 Solano Ave #546
Berkeley, CA 94707

Interior Design by Tabitha Lahr

She Writes Press is a division of SparkPoint Studio, LLC.
Company and/or product names that are trade names, logos, trademarks, and/or registered trademarks of third parties are the property of their respective owners and are used in this book for purposes of identification and information only under the Fair Use Doctrine.

Names and identifying characteristics have been changed to protect the privacy of certain individuals.

In memory of

Ivan Petrov
Beloved father, Chernobyl hero,
and accordion virtuoso

Galyna Petrova
Beloved babushka and songbird
of survival and mirth

"The stars we are given.
The constellations we make."

—REBECCA SOLNIT

Contents

Author's Note

This story of love and peacemaking begins after the fall of the Soviet Union and before Russia's twenty-first-century invasion of Ukraine. At that time, the Iron Curtain was wavering in shifting winds, allowing light to begin to penetrate its shadows. Democracy was taking root in Ukraine. Belarus, under the rule of an autocrat, had opened doors to outsiders. It was my good fortune to slip through that portal and witness the expansion. Anything—even a peaceful coexistence among the freed republics—seemed possible to me, a woman raised in the United States during the Cold War.

During this period, Russia's imprint on the other former republics remained evident, a red thread woven through a complex, ever-evolving tapestry of history, nuance, and cultures. It was still commonplace in casual conversation to refer to the people, foods, and customs of former Soviet republics as Russian. Some of the Ukrainians and Belarusians I came to know and love as a Children of Chernobyl volunteer engaged in this practice, though they identified first and foremost with the land and culture of their ancestors.

Zoya's Gift mirrors my experience and perspective of this complex intersection of languages and cultures. My apologies for any errors caused by my limited knowledge, particularly in languages and my still-evolving understanding of my cultural blind spots. In my efforts to be clear and accurate, I enlisted the guidance of a sensitivity reader, a Slavic language scholar, and copy editors. Since my trip to Ukraine, many street names and other words have been changed from Russian to Ukrainian spellings; I have tried to use the spellings that were in use at the time I was there.

To protect the privacy of the citizens of Belarus and Ukraine who appear in this story, all of their names, the names of villages where they live, and other identifying factors have been changed. The dialogues in this story were re-created to the best of my ability. However, due to translation misunderstandings and memory lapses, they may not reflect the precise meaning intended by the speakers and should not be considered direct quotations.

This memoir is based on my own subjective recollections, perspectives, and journal entries. Where I have filled in the gaps of memory, my intention was to capture my emotional truth. My hope is that the story rings true for everyone portrayed in these pages, despite our differences of culture, nationality, and language.

✦ Prologue

Standing on the aft deck of the *Kittitas* ferry, Michael and I watched the Seattle skyline disappear as we sailed across Puget Sound toward snow-capped mountains on the Olympic Peninsula. On that dazzling Friday afternoon in April 1986, clouds parted in the south and Mount Rainier took center stage, dressed in snow white and hints of blue ice.

Feeling safe and at home in the arms of my future husband, I drew in a deep breath of crisp salt air. We were on our way to the Boat Shed, the Bremerton restaurant where we'd gone to dinner on our first date.

"A perfect day," I said. It was the first anniversary of the day we'd met.

We didn't know about the nuclear disaster then unfolding in the Soviet Union. Nor about the cloud of radiation headed our way from the Chernobyl Nuclear Power Station in Ukraine.

As catastrophe struck on the other side of the world, Michael and I enjoyed the Boat Shed's food, mellow ambiance, and classic Northwest decor: Wood beams throughout. Floor-to-ceiling windows overlooking the water. White linen tablecloths and napkins adding a touch of elegance suited to our special occasion.

After finishing our celebratory dinner, we ferried back to Seattle in the moonlight. Lights twinkled from a necklace of homes and cottages lining the shores. The Space Needle hovered over the north end of downtown like a flying saucer. High-rise buildings stood out like a collection of illuminated Tinkertoy sculptures.

Cuddled together next to a window, Mike turned to me and smiled. In his gentle eyes, I saw a radiant and wise old soul gazing back at me, and I knew this man would walk with me to eternity. I couldn't yet see the heartbreak of infertility and the three pregnancy losses we would endure, or the impact that toxic chemicals would have on my health. And I couldn't yet know that the explosion of Chernobyl would spark to life a dream that had been gestating in me since childhood.

Part One:
Dreams

CHAPTER 1

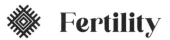 Fertility

1996

The heartbeat in my womb had disappeared like a falling star. Too stunned to cry or speak, I lay on the examination table in silence. Sitting in a chair beside me, Mike reached for my hand and wrapped his fingers around mine. I couldn't meet his eyes. I didn't want his heart to break when he saw the hollow shell that was now me.

"We need to go," my husband said softly, breaking the silence.

In slow motion I sat up, shifted my weight, and dropped my legs over the side of the table like a ninety-year-old woman barely able to move. Without looking, I knew sorrow shadowed his face and his brows were tight knots of despair. Still, I never doubted he would find the strength to walk me through the dark tunnel we had entered together. He was a man who didn't run from hard work or pain. Already he had lived up to the promises he had made in my darkest hours after our previous miscarriages. "It's you and me," he told me every day with both his words and his actions. "We'll get through this together. You're not alone." I knew he was solid loyalty and love.

Mike helped me get dressed and then opened the door. Side by side, we walked along the corridor. Nurses, doctors, and patients preoccupied with their own dramas passed by without making eye contact. We were invisible. In the lobby sat women with stony faces, leafing through magazines, waiting to be called in for sonograms, X-rays, and diagnoses that would send them on their way elated, reassured, terrified, or devastated. We made our way to the elevator, down to the basement parking garage, and into our car. With each step, I felt as though I were a ghost pushing through deep water.

After our two previous miscarriages, we had endured thirty-six months of extensive charting, invasive tests, and drugs with potential long-term consequences. All with no results. When I passed the age of forty, we decided to stop trying. The risk of another loss or an unhealthy baby seemed like more than we could bear. My life force was a tiny ember almost extinguished. Getting out of bed was an accomplishment. I knew it was time for us to end that horrible chapter of our lives and create a new story. But how? After three years of the all-consuming project of chasing pregnancy, I could not imagine a replacement for that vision. Grief tethered itself to me every waking hour. Life was slipping through my fingers.

My world was also shrinking, because I suffered from multiple chemical sensitivity (MCS), an environmental illness that causes physical, psychological, and emotional reactions to neurotoxic chemicals found in ordinary products considered to be safe. Exposures to perfume, scented lotions and deodorizers, dryer sheets, fresh paint, cleaning products, new carpet, or car exhaust impaired my cognitive functioning. I couldn't form coherent sentences to express my thoughts. I lost my balance, and experienced debilitating confusion, dizziness, exhaustion, headaches, and emotions.

To make my experience even more difficult, most doctors didn't—and still don't—recognize MCS as a physical illness, even though studies show brain function impairment induced by perfume and pesticide exposures. Those studies might explain, at least partially, how I developed MCS, infertility, and depression. When I grew up on a farm in Michigan in the 1950s, pesticides were considered miracle products used to increase crop yields and income with no harmful side effects on humans. My father had no idea he was saturating our environment with carcinogens, neurotoxic chemicals, and hormone disrupters when he sprayed our fields.

The only MCS treatment known to be effective was to avoid exposures. Given that almost no uncontaminated place existed in the world, it wasn't easy. I hated to tell people, especially friends and family, I couldn't be in their company unless they were unscented. Some people understood and were accommodating. Others felt resentful and controlled and couldn't manage to be scent-free. Still others became hostile. The only way to protect myself was to shrink my social world.

Living in a dark bubble filled with dread and hopelessness, I tried to dig my way out but couldn't make headway. In desperation, I took the advice of a doctor who encouraged me to take an antidepressant medication. "Just until you have a foundation under you again." Slowly but surely, the unbearable weight pressing down on me began to lift. At that point I discovered a book, *Sweet Grapes: How to Stop Being Infertile and Start Living Again*, written by a couple, both medical doctors, who had also experienced unsuccessful infertility treatment. Like Mike and me, they had ruled out adoption and other ways of building a family. In the book, they shared the process that had helped them embrace a child-free life as a family of two. The first step, they wrote, was to use birth control to solidify the decision and stop the obsessive thoughts that come with the possibility of pregnancy. After two miscarriages and months of unsuccessful fertility treatments, that step seemed unnecessary, if not ludicrous, so we ignored that recommendation.

Our process of healing and rediscovering the sweetness of intimacy with no other agenda had just begun when I realized I was pregnant for the third time. To say that I felt elated would not be truthful. In reality, I felt devastated. The unknown risks to the fetus from the antidepressant I was taking, especially in the first critical weeks of development, terrified me. I stopped taking the drug immediately. By the time that faint heartbeat faded away, my hormones and serotonin level were in free fall. I felt physically, emotionally, and psychologically wrecked.

This was our third miscarriage in the eight years we'd been married, the only pregnancy that had produced a pulsing heart on the ultrasound screen. Now, my body would purge or reabsorb the ashes of that tiny dream, wiping it out as though it never happened.

Mike drove to the exit, paid for the parking, then merged into the busy street as the parking attendant called out, "Have a nice day!" In my mind I screamed, but there was no sound. It was all I could do just to breathe. Mike and I both knew this marked the end of the fertility trail for us.

Still lost in a wilderness of grief and depression a year later, sitting in front of the television, I found myself drawn into a story about the Children of Chernobyl Northwest, a nonprofit organization that brought children from the former Soviet Union to Seattle for summer reprieves from radiation exposure. The reporter explained that the children's immune systems were compromised and many of the kids would develop thyroid cancer by the time they were teenagers.

Featured on the program was a seven-year-old girl from Belarus, the former Soviet Republic where the majority of the nuclear fallout from the Chernobyl explosion had landed. Seeing that vulnerable little girl with a triangle scarf covering her bald head struck a deep chord in me. It was obvious to me that I resonated with her suffering from an environmental illness, and obvious, too, that I yearned to comfort and care for a child. But I sensed there was something more, a stirring I couldn't yet explain, almost imperceptible, yet strong enough to push me to my feet to grab a notepad and pen. *Children of Chernobyl NW.* I wrote the name on a sheet of fresh white paper before it could disappear in a fog of depression. The next day I contacted the organization. That single phone call set me on a course that would transform my vision of motherhood and awaken a dormant Cold War dream to build a human bridge for peace.

CHAPTER 2

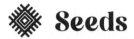 **Seeds**

The ground of that dormant childhood dream lay in Gratiot County, Michigan, on the farm where I was raised from infancy to adolescence.

The air felt thick with fear when I was growing up. Every night, I fell asleep to the background drone of Walter Cronkite's deep, steady voice delivering the news on the television. *Khrushchev. Communists. Fallout shelters. Nuclear warheads. Cuban Crisis. Russian missiles.* The tone of serious danger wormed its way into me, over and over. As a result, I became conditioned to believe that the Russians were plotting to kill us.

My mother was an anxious woman, always on guard. By the time I was seven years old, I knew that bankers were greedy men just waiting to take our Midwest farm in foreclosure and that strangers might be thieves, escaped convicts, or kidnappers. As a sensitive young girl, I could tell when Mom smelled danger by the way her body spoke. Her eyes narrowed. Arms stiffened. Spine straightened. I could feel her tension in my belly. Whenever my father was away, Mom slept with a pellet gun under her pillow and a shotgun at her side. "Just in case," she said.

Seeing those guns made my stomach turn queasy. Though it was unlikely that any violent criminals lurked nearby, I couldn't have known that. I shook with terror one night when, after hearing a noise outside, Mom crept to a window in full frontier mode, her trigger finger poised. My stomach rose to my throat. I never doubted she would shoot those guns. I'd seen her stand up to bankers who tried to bully her. With a sharp tongue, one eyebrow cocked, and her red-tinted lips pumping iron, she was a woman who couldn't be intimidated.

Mom's tension became my own. I grew up feeling unsafe and longed for a world attuned to love instead of fear. I charted a path in my heart, one that didn't require me to arm myself or to live in terror. My dream was to build a human bridge of peace between the United States and our so-called enemies behind the Iron Curtain. I was a girl who attended a one-room country school, swam in a gravel pit, and had never traveled outside our state, yet, somehow, I sensed that an emotional resonance could melt the iceberg between us and the Soviets. That seed would gestate in me for more than forty years.

My family didn't know any Russians. Mostly English and Germans farmed in Gratiot County. There wasn't much diversity in our neck of the woods, except during the summer months when Spanish-speaking migrant workers came up from Texas to weed our fields. Though I never heard a disparaging word spoken about those men whose skin was brown, I knew the unspoken rules that governed their behavior: *Stay out of the farmer's yard. Don't speak to his children. Bring your own water.*

Though the unspoken rules taught me to fear dark-skinned strangers, I felt drawn to these people whose language sounded like soft drumrolls to me. Contrary to my usual shy and wary self, I played on the junk pile behind our garage so I could hear conversations in Spanish while the men dug milkweeds and dandelions close by.

"*¿Cómo está tu familia?*" How is your family?

"*¡Muy bien! ¡Mi esposa tendrá un bebé pronto!*" Very good. My wife will have the baby soon.

The musical sound of their language and the freedom to indulge my curiosity from a close but "safe" distance thrilled me, though I never would have dared move any closer.

On Saturday nights, when the migrant families gathered in the churchyard across the road, I watched in fascination from behind our living room curtains. If I could travel back in time, I'd encourage my younger self to cross that road and express her desire to know their hearts and stories, to experience the thrill of communicating a simple "hello" in a new language. It sounds so easy now. Back then, taking such a risk was inconceivable and would have provoked a terrible scolding from my parents. Those were lines you didn't cross, lines that still exist for too many.

I didn't put it together then, but now I realize that the longing I felt to interact with people whose language and skin color were different from mine was an early sign. I couldn't have known as a child that I would require the richness and diversity of cross-cultural relationships to feel connected to the world.

It wouldn't have occurred to me or my parents that the Spanish-speaking migrants were descendants of indigenous peoples native to the continent. Years would pass before I would begin to understand the complexities of the fact that in the United States, a country founded on slavery and genocide, the perceived enemy too often feared by white people had dark skin, dark hair, and dark eyes. In truth, *we* were the colonizers, the ones to be feared. Though the men weeding our fields must have carried that truth like thorns in their eyes, they showed no disrespect.

Years later, as I struggled to heal from the heartbreak of three lost pregnancies, the time came for me to manifest the bridge of my childhood dream. It was a perfect spring day in the Pacific Northwest. Fiddleheads were poking out of sword ferns, rhododendron buds were bursting with magenta flowers, and a great blue heron winged past the house when Nadya, the Children of Chernobyl coordinator, called to confirm that two eight-year-old girls from Zalessie, a village in Belarus, would be spending the summer with Mike and me.

"Twins!" she announced.

A jolt of emotion shot through me. *Twins!* The word splashed in my heart. The fantasy of parenting twins had taken hold of me as a child, when I saw Hayley Mills, then a young movie star, playing dual roles as twins in *The Parent Trap*, my favorite Walt Disney film. Those mischievous little blonde-haired imps had so captivated me that I longed to mother twins one day. That fantasy had stuck. My chances had seemed good, given that on my mother's side of the family were two sets of twins. I had prayed for twins each time I conceived.

Now, my whole body buzzed with shock, joy, and grief. Goose bumps rose on my arms. I knew this moment couldn't be explained by coincidence or serendipity. Feeling swept up by the mysteries of kismet, I could hardly focus on the details Nadya provided.

The twins' father, she explained, had been employed at the power station at the time of the disaster and returned to Chernobyl as a liquidator—one of the 500,000 crewmen deployed to clean up the radioactive debris in the wake of the explosion. Their parents, both Ukrainian, and their older sister had been resettled in Belarus, where over 60 percent of the nuclear fallout had landed. The twins were born there two years later, under that cloud of radiation.

"They don't speak any English," the coordinator informed me. In Belarus, Russian was (and still is) the primary language.

"I'll send you a handout with a few Russian words and phrases that might come in handy," she promised.

Growing up on a farm in the American Midwest, everything I knew about the Soviet Union I learned from daily newscasts on the black-and-white TV that sat in the corner of our living room. In my mind, the USSR was synonymous with Russia, a frightening one-dimensional wall of missiles, spies, onion domes, and danger. The US government's propaganda campaigns during the Cold War had reduced those millions of people from fifteen republics to one simple construct known as "The Enemy."

Only years later would I learn that the USSR was a collection of republics held together by a treaty, and that the differences between these unique cultures became muddled when Russia imposed its language and a single nationalism. Ukraine and Belarus wouldn't fully register on my internal map of the world until I opened my heart and home to strangers from these intertwined countries.

Now, my mind spun, trying to put together the pieces of a confusing new puzzle of people, places, and cultures that were foreign to me. As I tried to picture the girls, Ukrainian by descent, Belarusian by birth, and Russian by culture, I realized I had no clear image of what they might look like. I had a pretty clear picture of a person from Italy or Sweden. But my mind drew a blank when it came to Russians, Ukrainians, and Belarusians.

Without yet understanding how my experience as an American had influenced my impressions, or realizing I was projecting my internalized idea of "the enemy," I began to picture the twins coming my way with dark hair and mysterious dark eyes.

My heart overflowed with the gratitude and joy of feeling a prayer had been answered, not as I had pictured, but in a soul-satisfying way I couldn't have imagined.

Part Two:
1997

CHAPTER 3

✸ Two Little Girls and One Small Duffel

Buzzing with excitement on the day of the twins' arrival, I heated the oven. Lined up on my kitchen counter were glass canning jars and all the ingredients for preparing a dish I called "Russian Chicken": a heap of chicken thighs and drumsticks, sliced onions, dozens of peeled garlic cloves, prunes, dried apricots, golden raisins, a mound of salt and another of pepper. I coated each piece of chicken with a generous pinch of the salt and pepper and packed them in the jars with layers of the dried fruits, onions, and garlic.

Falling-off-the-bones tender and scrumptious, this dish, introduced to me by an artist from Moscow living in San Francisco, had become my signature dinner for special occasions. I assumed it would be familiar to the Belarusian girls who would soon be sitting at my table, and certain they would be famished after their long journey to Seattle. With half a dozen quart jars filled to the brim, there would be more than enough to feed a family of twelve. As my mother's daughter, I felt compelled to go overboard when it came to food and guests. And this occasion certainly called for celebration. Though I was a seasoned host to friends and family, including special visits with nieces and nephews who came from out of state for a week or two without their parents, I was stepping into a new role outside my comfort zone. The moment felt pregnant with purpose I couldn't yet fully understand. I was birthing a dream, and in just a few short hours I would be mothering twins.

Before Mike and I headed to the airport to meet the twins, I covered each jar with a square of tinfoil and set them in the oven to bake. By the time we returned, a heavenly nectar of juices would be bubbling furiously, the chicken ready to be served on a heap of mashed potatoes, also made in advance, and topped with a dollop of sour cream mixed with lemon juice.

At SeaTac Airport, a crush of people stood waiting outside customs. Threads of conversation unspooled in many languages. Dizzying scents of hair tonic, cloves, and perspiration wafted through the cavernous hall.

Overwhelmed by the fragrances and nervous anticipation, I held Mike's hand as we maneuvered through the crowd in search of the local Children of Chernobyl coordinator. Finally, I spotted Nadya, a tiny woman with long brown hair, heavy bangs, and a calm demeanor. We joined the cluster of host parents surrounding her. Together we waited for the two dozen children and their chaperone to arrive on a flight from Moscow.

Banter skidded around the group like a polka, filled with the thrill and confidence of experienced parents and volunteer hosts. As the only first-timers in the group, and with no parenting experience under our belts, Mike and I listened and smiled but said little. We knew almost nothing about Belarus before we'd signed up as host parents and had no idea what to expect with children under our wings who couldn't speak or understand a word of English. Apprehension tinged our excitement.

The energy in our midst whipped into a froth when the Aeroflot flight touched down. After an agonizing wait, a wave of passengers began forming queues at customs stations separated from us by a glass wall.

"There they are!" cried a woman in our group.

I rose to the tips of my toes, trying to spot two young look-alike girls. I saw only a confusion of strangers until I noticed a young boy exiting a queue with his passport in hand. He raced to the window wall and stood, earnestly peering through the glass to find a familiar face in the crowd. The host mother standing beside me raised her arm and waved wildly.

"Here! Over here!" A tear slid down her cheek.

Suddenly, the boy's face lit like a torch and his arms flew up over his head. Though we couldn't hear him, his gaping smile and busy lips told me he was yipping and yelling with glee.

One by one, a string of kids formed a line on either side of the boy. Bundles of energy fueled by adrenaline, they danced like jumping beans as they waited until the whole group was cleared and they could exit customs. The line kept growing. Whoops of joy erupted on both sides of the glass each time a child made eye contact with their host parents. These children felt safe venturing to the other side. No Iron Curtain stood between us.

My body tingled with pins and needles when the customs doors slid open and the children poured out like water tumbling over boulders. Our circle expanded as families reunited with their beloved Belarusian kids in a flood of tears, relief, and long embraces. The chaperone, Victor, a tall man with a balding crown and a fist full of documents, positioned himself in the middle of our tribe. Straining to be heard above the din, he called out host family names and matched each one with the appropriate child's paperwork. One by one, the families claimed the forms and rushed away with the Belarusian child they had dearly missed for months. As the hall cleared, my heart began to sink. Had the twins been unable to make the trip?

After all the other children were claimed and gone, Victor bellowed, "Michael and Gail McCormick!" I raised my hand.

"That's us!"

Only then did I become aware of two girls huddled beside him as though glued to his legs. Except for big, black circles of sleep deprivation surrounding their eyes, and butterscotch-colored hair cut chin length, there were few similarities between them. One was a tall wisp with frightened green eyes. The other one, with a round face and inquisitive blue-green eyes, stood several inches shorter. Pushing them toward us, Victor introduced the apprehensive twins.

"Maria Petrova," he said, putting one hand on the shoulder of the taller girl. "And Vika Petrova." He placed his other hand on the shorter twin.

The airport chaos faded out of my awareness. My mommy genes kicked into gear, and I kneeled in front of the eight-year-old twins. "Hello," I said, keeping my voice low and even. I handed a stuffed monkey with long, wiggly arms and legs to Vika.

"*Spacibo*," she mumbled, tucking the monkey under her arm. *Thank you*. Without speaking another word, she kept her eyes trained on me, recording every nuance, as I turned my attention to Maria.

"I'm Gail," I said, handing a monkey to the taller girl. Maria's eyes caught mine briefly, then quickly darted away.

"*Spacibo*," she croaked.

"This is Mike," I said, making room for him to kneel beside me.

"Hello. Welcome," said Mike softly, though usually his voice boomed like a radio announcer's.

Too shocked to feel much of anything and unable to understand English, neither girl broke a smile. Travel with friends was over. Half a planet away from their mama and papa, they were going home with strangers. With the brief introduction completed, the chaperone handed us the girls' medical documents and waved us off with no instructions, no user manual, not even a "good luck!" Even the local coordinator had already left. The informality struck me as inadequate considering the level of responsibility we were undertaking.

Momentarily frozen, I caught Mike's eye. In his gaze I saw the reassuring confidence of a many-faceted man who wore suits and ties and robin's-egg-blue buttoned-down shirts, carried a briefcase, mentored young colleagues, managed investments, and produced reports. His head was filled with facts and figures, but his heart overflowed with love and patient perseverance. I traced with my eyes the three lines etched into his brow—one for every miscarriage he had seen me through. I'd learned he had the capacity for happiness on any path as long as I was happy. This was my dream coming to life, and he was in 100 percent. At that moment there was nothing more important to him than the two girls in our care. And I saw the father he might have been.

Knowing my husband had my back, I took a deep breath. We each took the hand of a girl and made our way to the baggage area. My thoughts scrambled. *How in the world will we make it through a silent thirty-minute drive home, not to mention the rest of the summer?* We had studied Russian for beginners but struggled with the Cyrillic alphabet and accents. Besides a few basic words, nothing had stuck.

Smiling, I made my way through the airport like I knew what I was doing. One little black duffel sat on the baggage carousel. The girls recognized it right away. By American standards, it seemed so small for two girls. I didn't want to leave a bag behind, so, by scrunching my eyebrows into question marks, pointing to the bag, and holding up two fingers, I tried to ask the girls if they had brought a second one. To my delight, Vika understood my question. She shook her head no. Our first attempt to communicate was successful. *Yes!*

At the car, Mike and I buckled the girls into the back seat. After their twelve-hour bus ride from Minsk to Moscow and a ten-hour flight to Seattle, they could hardly keep their eyes open as we zipped onto the freeway in a world completely foreign to them.

"You must be tired," I said gently, turning toward the back seat, wanting to comfort them. Maria stared at me like a zombie, but a hint of curiosity registered in Vika's eyes. I took this as a good omen, one that gave me a little hope that Mike and I weren't in water too deep for us.

On the viaduct above the waterfront in downtown Seattle, I tried again to ease the awkwardness for the girls. "Ferry boat!" I said, pointing out the window at the vessel crossing Puget Sound. But the girls' faces remained blank, their eyes vacant. I might as well have said, "Welcome to Mars." It was ridiculous, of course, to think that they might understand what I was pointing at. But I couldn't just be quiet. My mind kept searching for a way to make them feel safe and comfortable.

Unable to think of anything else to say or do, I turned my attention to their medical documents, written in a confusing mix of Russian and English, in tiny print. One part I could decipher listed medical conditions preceded by a box that was checked if the child had been diagnosed with that condition. What I saw alarmed me.

"Oh no! One of them is a bed wetter!" I said, now grateful that the girls couldn't understand a word I said. Unable to tell which document went with which girl, I turned to study the two of them in the back seat.

"It must be Maria," I concluded. She appeared scrawny and unwell, as though she might vomit at any moment. Alarm bells screeched in my head, and my imagination began to run amok. *What if she has a serious condition we're not equipped to handle?*

"You'll have to run out and buy a plastic sheet to cover the mattress," I told Mike. "But wait until after we've eaten. And don't let the girls see it when you bring it home. I don't want them to feel embarrassed or ashamed."

Another anxious question hit me just as Mike parked the car at the curb in front of our 1950s Roman brick house. *What if the twins are disappointed to find themselves part of a family with no swing set, no pets, and no American siblings to play with?* Determined to create a summer of delights the girls would remember fondly, I pushed that question away, glad we had volunteered to host two children so they could be playmates.

"*Dome!*" I announced, using one of the few Russian words I remembered. *Home.*

We piled out of the car and led the girls up the stairs to the front door. Welcomed by the sweet and savory scents of garlic, chicken, and fruit, we wound our way through the kitchen to the guest room. On the bed lay two blue-denim jumpers and two striped T-shirts, one pink and one yellow, that I'd bought for the girls.

Looking back, I would realize that denim clothes were about as close to US uniforms as one could get, the ultimate symbol of rugged American individualism. And I would understand this flagged the beginning of my conflict of presenting America to the girls.

"For you!" I said, pointing to the clothes.

Sitting on the bed with their duffel placed between them, the girls sprang to life but ignored the clothes I'd bought for them. A gleam appeared in Maria's eyes. Vika's cheeks turned the color of peaches. Together, they pulled on the duffel's zipper and the bag sprang open. Like two magicians pulling an endless scarf from a hat, they reached in and began to pull out a stream of gifts they'd brought for Mike and me. Our jaws dropped as the girls, now confident and self-possessed, presented us with candy, cut glass, table linens, ceramic bowls, and vodka. This was our introduction to their customary gift-giving ritual.

Last, the twins unpacked their most precious cargo—a family photo album. Maria opened it to a picture of their family posed in front of a gray one-story house trimmed with blue window frames, white diamond motifs, and a corrugated tin roof. Wrapped in heavy coats, the family was dressed for winter. In the background, an accordion sat on the ground near a bottle that had been tossed away. An old bicycle lay on its side.

Vika pointed to a gray-haired woman seated on an old bench, a headscarf tied under her chin. "*Eto* Babushka." *This is Grandma.*

"Papa's mama?" Mike asked.

"*Da.*" *Yes.*

Over time, we would learn that the house in the picture belonged to Babushka and was located in a Ukrainian village, built for Chernobyl survivors, where she and her husband had resettled after they were evacuated from the contaminated area.

I pointed to the young girl draped across Babushka's lap. "*Eto* Maria?"

"*Da,*" Maria answered.

Vika then pointed to a woman who appeared to be in her midthirties, short dark hair framing her face. "*Eto* Mama," she said.

"Ah, your mama!" I responded. "My name is Gail, your name is Vika," I said, pointing first to myself then to her.

"Your mama's name?" I asked, pointing to her in the picture. Vika scrunched her eyebrows in confusion. I watched her trying to connect the dots. Suddenly her face brightened and she sat up straight.

"Zoya!" she answered.

"Mama's name is Zoya?"

"*Da!*"

"This is Vika?" Mike asked, pointing to the young girl leaning into Zoya in the picture.

"*Da.*"

As we huddled over the photo album with our heads bumping and arms touching, we were introduced to the others in the photograph—the twins' papa, Ivan; their older sister, Elina; and cousins. From my American view, I wouldn't have guessed they were warm, fun-loving people. Elina smiled for the camera, but the rest of the family appeared dour and grim. Yet the twins' comfort with physical contact and the joy I heard in their voices each time they spoke of their kin conveyed to me that, underneath the fatigue and shock, these girls were no strangers to warmth and affection. Later I would learn that in their culture people didn't normally smile for photos. In fact, people who smiled for no obvious reason were considered foolish. This was just one of many surprises in store for me and Mike, a guy known for his quick and sometimes cheesy smile.

After meeting their family through photographs, we unpacked the clothes they'd brought for the summer—an extra set of play clothes, a Sunday-best dress, and an extra pair of underwear. Through the eyes of a Westerner, it seemed like so little. I automatically began creating a mental list of things they would "need."

In the bottom of the bag Zoya had tucked in a letter she had handwritten in Cyrillic to Mike and me. In the letter, translated several days later, Zoya expressed both concern and gratitude. "They are good girls, but sometimes they can be mischievous," she wrote. "I hope you understand and that they will be polite and help you with your work."

After we had emptied the duffel, I turned my attention to dinner. "Are you hungry?" I asked Vika and Maria, patting my stomach and raising my voice an octave at the end of my sentence to indicate it was a question. They understood immediately.

"*Da!*" the twins replied in unison. Nodding their heads, they took their seats in the dining room. Their eyes grew wide when I placed a large bowl heaped with chicken thighs and drumsticks in the middle of the table.

"*Russkiy* chicken!" I announced proudly, certain the twins would find the food both delicious and familiar. Their instant laughter utterly confused me. While trying to imagine why they might think I'd made a joke, I continued to smile. Did they think I was suggesting the chicken had come from Russia? Was President Lukashenko the only person in Belarus who could afford a pile of meat on his plate? This was just one of many moments of confusion and unanswered questions we would encounter in the unavoidable gaps created by our language and cultural differences.

Mike dropped big globs of potato on the girls' plates and covered them with the chicken concoction. They took turns spooning sour cream on top and dug into the food.

"*Vkusno,*" said Maria. I had no idea the word meant *tasty.*

"*Ya nye ponimayu,*" I responded. *I don't understand.*

"*Koos-na!*" she repeated, raising her volume in case I was hearing impaired.

"I'm so sorry," I apologized again, still clueless.

With increasing frustration, she repeated herself several more times. When it finally dawned on her that I wouldn't understand even if she tried a hundred times, she gave up and finished her meal in forlorn silence. Helpless, I apologized again for my ignorance. How could we ever develop a relationship with these girls if we couldn't talk to each other?

As the twins devoured everything on their plates and gladly accepted second helpings, my concerns diminished. If nothing else, the language of food would convey love and carry us through the summer.

It would be several weeks before their appetites tapered off. Between them, they guzzled an entire gallon of apple juice every two days and rapidly devoured bananas, grapes, and other fruits. We learned this pattern was normal, because fresh fruits and vegetables were scarce in Belarus. Cabbage and tomatoes, staples in their culture, were the only vegetables they would eat unless we bribed them with ice cream. Most foods they preferred smothered in mayonnaise or ketchup, which they referred to as *sauce*. They wouldn't allow ground beef to touch their plates, let alone their lips. You would've thought we were trying to force them to consume old hockey pucks, not hamburgers. Chicken, fish, and hot dogs—*sausage*—were the big hits.

With their tummies full, the twins' eyelids could hardly stay open. Mike went to shop for a plastic bedsheet while I drew a bath for the girls. When hot, steamy water gushed out of the faucet into the tub, they giggled with delight. I would learn that they were accustomed to a slow drizzle of hot water during winter months and periods of no hot water during summer utilities maintenance.

While the girls chattered in the tub, I went to the kitchen to review their medical documents one more time. That's when I realized my mistake. The checked box was for a digestive disorder, not bed-wetting. Just as that realization hit me, Mike walked in holding up a bag containing the plastic sheet, success written across his face.

"False alarm!" I cheerfully announced. "She's not a bed wetter after all!"

Mike's face drooped. He shot me a look that said, *Why didn't you figure that out before I went out?* Then he shrugged and tossed the bag on a chair. "I can take this back tomorrow," he said. "Where are the girls?"

"Still in the tub."

"Have you checked on them?"

"Several times. They're fine, but if I let them stay in the water much longer, they'll shrivel up and turn into miniature *babushkas.*"

"Can't hurt 'em. Might as well let them enjoy it as long as they're happy."

Those long, leisurely baths became a nightly ritual. Shamelessly, before the summer ended, I served the girls apple juice or 7UP in the tub, at their request. Though princess treatment ran counter to what I considered appropriate parental behavior, I couldn't help myself. How could I refuse them when they felt so comfortable, like members of the family, that they weren't afraid to ask? I didn't care that I was being played.

Wrapped in the thick cotton bath towels I'd left out for them, the girls emerged at last. Then, while I blew Vika's hair dry with an electric dryer attached to the bathroom wall, Maria sat on the vanity counter waiting for her turn. With the residue of their long journey washed away and their hunger sated, they happily surrendered to my pampering.

Next, I presented them with new Disney toothbrushes and dental floss. As host parents, we were encouraged to arrange for the children to receive dental examinations, cleanings, and necessary treatment, and to instill in them the importance of consistent dental hygiene, which wasn't a priority in their culture.

"Very good!" I remarked as the girls pulled the waxed floss in and out between their teeth. Then, ready for sleep, they slipped into the double bed they were to share. Mike and I tucked them in with a kiss on the cheek.

"*Spokonoy nochi*," I whispered. *Good night.*

"*Spokonoy nochi*," said two tiny voices.

Next door, in our bedroom adjacent to the girls', Mike and I lay together as the summer sky slowly darkened.

"They're so little!" I whispered. "I hope they're not scared. I'm keeping both bedroom doors open so I can hear if either one wakes up crying in the night."

"Their mama and papa have put a lot of trust in us," said Mike. "I can't imagine having my kid going to bed in a stranger's house with no way to contact them."

"I love having their hearts in our house," I said, drifting off to sleep.

At 7:00 a.m. I awakened to birdsong. The house felt still and quiet, as though Mike and I were home alone. Turning over, I asked him, "Are there really two little girls sleeping in the room next to ours?" Though his eyes were still closed, he smiled.

"Let's go see."

Expecting to find them sleeping, we peeked into the guest room. My heart leaped when I saw the twins sitting on the bed, dressed in their new T-shirts and denim jumpers, patiently waiting to explore a new world. The sheets had already been pulled tight, the pillows fluffed and skillfully placed along the headboard. Their faces shone with openness and anticipation.

"*Dobroye utro!*" Mike greeted them. *Good morning.*

"Look at you two brave girls!" I said.

Though the morning was already hot and muggy, they wore over their jumpers the heavy sweaters they'd brought from home, like little security blankets.

CHAPTER 4

❖ Creating a Mother Tongue

Side by side, the twins twirled in the swivel chairs parked in front of the living room window. Vika's brushed hair gleamed. Maria's hair was skewed in every direction. Seaplanes buzzed overhead, flying north toward the San Juan Islands. Boats zipped across Puget Sound, headed to the Hiram Chittenden Locks. Sea lions barked in the distance.

Mike and I were in the kitchen, cleaning up after breakfast. "Why don't we take them swimming in Lake Washington?" I suggested. "The host parents I talked to at the airport said all the kids from Belarus love to swim."

"Good idea," he said. "What are we going to do about bathing suits?"

"No problem," I assured him. "We'll stop at Fred Meyer on the way." A recent addition to our neighborhood, Fred Meyer resembled an old-fashioned general store for the twenty-first-century. Under one roof, it carried everything from groceries and garden supplies to paint, furniture, electronics, and clothes. "What I don't know is how we're going to explain our plan to the girls."

"I've got this," Mike assured me. Dressed in cargo shorts and a wrinkled T-shirt, he headed from the kitchen to the living room spinning his arms like a swimmer.

"Can you swim? You like to swim?" he asked the girls. His arms crawled through the air in giant strokes. Watching him, I chuckled.

The twins' feet hit the floor to stop their chairs from whirling. Maria eyed Mike through a lock of disheveled hair dangling over her face. Vika squinted her eyes as though trying to correct her vision. Suddenly, a glimmer of understanding registered in Vika's eyes.

"*Da! Da!*" she cried. "*Plavat!*" she explained to Maria. *Swim.* Then Maria joined the chorus. "*Da!*" Their eyes twinkled.

"Zalessie *plavat?*" asked Mike, trying to verify that Vika and Maria had experience swimming at home.

"*Da!*" the girls assured him. I marveled that, already, we were communicating so well.

"Okay! Let's go!" Mike shouted like a cheerleader.

I motioned for the girls to follow me into the kitchen, and they danced along behind me. Feeling like a middle-aged Mary Poppins blown into a new adventure, I pulled juice boxes, cold cuts, bread, mayonnaise, and carrot sticks out of the refrigerator while Mike brought the cooler up from the garage. As I slapped sandwiches together and slipped them into plastic bags, the girls packed them into the old red-and-white ice chest sitting on the floor. Chattering in Russian, they purred with happiness until Vika's face turned dark and stern and she hissed at Maria.

"*Niet!*" Maria roared back. *No.* A red blush rose from her throat to her forehead. Her jaw was set tight.

Shocked by the sudden outburst, I put down my knife, still dripping with mayonnaise, and placed a gentle hand on each girl's shoulder. "No fight-ing!" I warbled like a three-note song.

With their mama's and papa's voices still fresh in their minds, telling them to be good and to mind Gail and Mike, they backed down. Like magic, Vika's face turned sunny; Maria began humming. Their work together resumed without another word. But they could maintain their best behavior for only so long. I would learn these quarrels erupted with surprising frequency and could explode like wildfire.

After the girls packed the last sandwich on ice and fastened the lid, they each gripped a handle and carried the cooler to the front door like an old treasure chest. They set it on the floor with exaggerated grunts and groans. Then, like soldiers guarding gold, Vika sat on the top and Maria stood beside her while Mike and I flew around the house gathering beach towels and filling an old, frayed wicker bag with hats, sunscreen, magazines, and bottles of water.

"Okay, *davay!*" Mike called out. *Come on.*

Vika jumped up and Maria dashed to the door, holding it open for Mike as he carried the cooler out to the car. Then she grabbed the wicker bag and lugged it down the stairs behind him with the sun bouncing off her smooth, shiny hair. Maria piled the stack of beach towels into her arms and started for the stairs with her eyes barely visible above the folds.

"Here, let me take some of those," I said, picturing her tumbling down the stairs. Planning to reduce her load enough to prevent a disaster from occurring before we left home, I reached for a towel. In response, Maria spoke her first two words of English.

"No! I!"

I hesitated. Was this a moment to insist on protecting, or a moment to support the independence of these little chicks? The determination I saw in Maria's eyes told me not to interfere.

"Okay," I said. "Careful!" My tone revealed more concern than I had intended.

I tugged on a lock of my hair as Maria approached the stairs. With her chin held up over the stack of towels, she began a slow descent. Carefully locating each stair with a searching foot, she reached the car without incident. I breathed a sigh of relief and raked my fingers through my short curls. After a last look around for anything we had missed, I hustled to the car.

Five minutes later, Mike parked at Fred Meyer. The girls and I rushed into the store. Though they didn't understand the purpose of our mission, I knew they would catch on soon. When we reached the children's department, I stopped to inspect a small collection of swimsuits hanging on a rack.

"This one?" I asked Vika, handing her a one-piece flower-bed of pink, orange, and blue. She took it with no remark.

"*Eto?*" I asked Maria, turning to her with a red suit I thought might fit her tall, thin frame. "Or *eto?*" I held up a polka-dotted option. She shrugged her shoulders.

Waving the girls along, I led them to a dressing room. The three of us crammed inside and closed the door. The girls pulled off their shorts and shirts and shimmied into the swimsuits.

"You like?" I nodded my head up and down as I held one thumb up. "Or *niet?*" I asked, shaking my head from side to side and pointing my thumb down.

Vika shot me a thumbs-up and a smile that made her eyes squint. Maria, wearing the red number, remained silent and pursed her lips.

"So-so?" I tilted my flat palm side to side.

Maria wagged her hand back and forth. "So-so," she repeated, her arm bent at the elbow.

"Okay. Try this one," I said, offering her the other option—lime green covered with orange polka dots. After she had pulled on the suit, she smiled at the mirror and raised her thumb.

"Okay! *Poshli!*" I responded. *Let's go.* A deep delight nestled into my heart.

The girls changed back into street clothes and we headed to the checkout. On the way, I stopped in front of a tower of children's sunglasses that caught my eye. The two girls began trying on the glasses, leaning in to see their reflections in the tiny mirror attached to the display rack. It didn't take Vika more than a minute to choose a model with oval lenses and red hearts on the frame. She was a girl who knew instantly what she wanted. Like me, Maria agonized over too many choices.

"Maria! *Pozhaluysta, davay!*" Vika begged, chafing to get to the beach. *Please. Come on.*

Under pressure, Maria finally settled on a rock star style—reflective silver-coated lenses. We lined up at the register, paid, then race-walked back to the car.

Mike put aside his *Sports Illustrated* and turned the key in the ignition. "You got swimsuits?" he asked.

"And sunglasses," I chirped.

His eyebrows rose. I wasn't sure if this meant *I get it* or *Isn't that a little over the top?* Our blue-collar roots had instilled caution in us when it came to spending money. Neither of us was overly materialistic by American standards. We shared an appreciation for a simple life. But we enjoyed a comfortable lifestyle that included vacations and sometimes purchasing non-essentials. I *wanted* to spoil the girls, and I knew Mike would too. But we were aware that our choices might impact these two young girls in ways we couldn't fully understand. Before their arrival, we had agreed that we wanted to share with them not only our resources but our value of moderation as well. We didn't want to leave them with the impression that the United States was one big Disneyland or set them up for excessive expectations. Somehow, we thought, we would find the right balance. But already that line was fuzzy for me.

While I clipped tags off the new purchases, we cruised up one hill and down the next, winding our way across Seattle to *Ozero* Washington. *Lake* Washington.

The water glistened. Sunbathers, towels, and blankets covered the long sandy beach. While Mike unpacked the car, I took the twins to the restroom to change into their new swimsuits. The air inside was thick with the aroma of discarded diapers, sand, and sunscreen. The girls observed the rows of stalls and turned to me for instructions. I pointed them toward two open doors.

Vika disappeared behind a door and slid the lock into place. "Maria! *Tualet!*" she announced. *Toilet.*

From behind the doors, she and Maria gleefully chatted while exploring their first public restroom in America. Their voices echoed off the walls. Rolls of toilet paper spun. The toilets flushed multiple times. Was this normal eight-year-old behavior, I wondered, or were these girls unaccustomed to lavatories with yards and yards of toilet paper? I thought about public restrooms I had encountered while traveling in Europe, where I had paid a small fee to receive a few squares of toilet paper before entering a stall.

Below the doors, I could see the girls stand on one leg, then the other, stepping out of their shorts and into the bathing suits. At last, they emerged, handing me their wadded-up clothes. I proceeded to show them how to activate the automatic water faucets and hand dryers, tasks they performed with exuberance.

"I go now," I said, pointing to myself, then to a stall. "You wait here," I added, pointing to them, then to the spot where they were standing. Then, I pointed to the door and shook my head left to right. "*Niet.* Don't leave without me." I didn't yet know they weren't likely to wander off alone.

While I changed my clothes, I heard in the background a symphony of water running intermittently, blow dryers kicking in repetitively, and a melody of Russian chatter. When I emerged in my swimsuit, the girls turned on the water and hand dryer for me as though waiting on royalty.

We found Mike waiting outside, eyes closed, cap on backward, face turned sunward. I broke his trance with a poke in the ribs. His eyes opened and telegraphed a question: *What in the world took you so long in there?*

"The toilets and faucets and hand dryers were pretty entertaining!" I explained. He shrugged his shoulders then picked up the cooler. Carrying all of our gear, our foursome trooped across the beach, dodging the patchwork of towels and blankets.

"How's this?" Mike asked, planting the cooler in the sand.

"Great!" I answered, happy to find a space where I didn't detect strong scents drifting our way. While I laid out our blankets, Mike turned to the girls.

"Okay, let's go!" he cried, leaning into a running stance as though he planned to race them. Kicking up sand, the girls took off with Mike chasing them.

To my surprise, Mike, a man who hated cold water, dove into the lake without hesitation. Normally he edged in, arms wrapped around himself while his body slowly made its peace with the frigid temperature.

Vika and Maria screeched with delight when Mike snuck up behind them underwater and grabbed their legs. Surfacing, he knitted his fingers together to form a cup and demonstrated how he could flip the girls into the air. Maria jumped in front of him, steadied herself with one hand on Mike's shoulder, and lifted her foot into the waiting container. Pinching her nose and screaming, she launched into the air and splashed down into the green water. Before she had surfaced, Vika scooted over to Mike and lifted her foot.

"I, Mike! I!" she squealed.

Then Maria begged for more. "Mike! Mike!"

Their trust in Mike amazed me, as did his ability to rev up his playful kid energy in spite of his full schedule of exhausting business trips and meetings. Over the years, I'd watched him making close connections with our nieces and nephews. He was an uncle who asked questions, drew them out, teased, encouraged, and comforted. Now I saw him bring that same loving presence to these children from outside our family circle. I loved him for that.

Vika spotted me standing at the shoreline. "Gail! Gail!" she called.

Smiling and waving, covered with sunscreen to protect my fair skin, I plunged in. As the initial shock of the cold wore off, I glided toward them, allowing the deep-green water to caress me. A contentment I hadn't felt in a long time seeped into my heart. A cacophony of children yelping, water splashing, babies crying, and dogs barking filled the air. Like a new mother attuned to her baby's cry, I could already tell which screeches were Maria's and Vika's, even with my eyes closed.

"Gail!" Maria called. Reaching for Mike, she wanted me to see her fly over his shoulder and into the waves.

"No, Mike tired," he told her.

"Yes, Mike! *Odin!*" she begged. *One.*

"*Odin*, Mike!" Vika chimed in.

"I think you need to do one more," I said, laughing.

"Okay, one more. *Odin.*"

I cheered as each girl sailed backward into the water one last time. Then I took the lead while Mike caught his breath. "Okay, come on!" I said, pushing off into a gentle side-stroke, kicking my pale white legs. Mike cruised beside me, enjoying the break from heavy lifting. Vika and Maria sputtered along behind us, spitting like happy clams. Though we stayed inside the ropes marking off the deep water, I kept a close eye on our girls. Dog-paddling as fast as they could, they kept pace with us, but their erratic course made me realize they weren't actually swimming. They were propelling themselves forward by pushing off from the sandy bottom, over and over, while furiously working their arms.

"I hope I've put on enough sunscreen," Mike said, momentarily distracting me from the twins.

"I hope so too. Your scalp is pink," I warned him.

A new chapter in our life had opened. Our eyes locked in sweet connection. Such moments hadn't come easily over the past few years of fertility treatments, pregnancy losses, and depression. I wanted to stretch this one out like hot saltwater taffy. I wanted it to stick. On the verge of losing myself in Mike's blue eyes, I glanced over my shoulder just in time to see the girls veering toward deep water.

"Mike! They can't swim!" I yelled, lunging toward them. We grabbed them just as the bottom disappeared from under their feet. Our fearless twins were sinking and choking, but that didn't dampen their spirits one iota. Still in full throttle, they merely changed course.

Life with our Belarusian twins presented constant surprises. One evening, I pulled out a children's card game that would be simple to teach them. To my delight, they recognized the game.

"UNO!" they cheered together.

Before you could say shazam, we were sitting around the big maple table like a bunch of old gaming geezers, shooting each other snarky glances and slapping cards down on the table so hard that the crystal rattled in the china cabinet against the wall. After a few rounds we were all bilingual players, able to switch from red to *krasnyy*, yellow to *zheltyy*, blue to *siniy*, and green to *zelenyi*, according to our whims. And Mike and I added a new sentence to our vocabulary: *Kukuruza pozhaluysta! Popcorn, please!*

But there were situations that begged for communication skills beyond our abilities. One of those was the evening we were out walking when, out of the blue, Maria asked us to tell people she was Indian.

"Indian?" I asked incredulously.

I didn't know if she meant Native American or East Indian, or what would motivate her to make such a request. I knew there must be something troubling her underneath it. Unable to have a conversation with her to explore her thoughts and feelings, I felt helpless. The impossibility of knowing what she needed made me so uncomfortable that I wanted to spin her request into a joke in order to relieve my pain. But I knew that would likely leave her to carry the burden of hurt or shame.

Maria giggled as though making light of her request. But she mustered up her courage. "Yes," she confirmed, avoiding eye contact.

"No Belarus?" I asked.

"No say Chernobyl," she answered softly.

Her response both surprised and saddened me. I had read that some misinformed Soviets had feared they could be contaminated from close contact with Chernobyl survivors. Others didn't believe they had suffered any real consequences and didn't deserve special treatment by the government or nonprofit groups. Soviet officials downplayed the physical effects of radiation exposure and suggested that worry and fear were the greatest threats.

Did Maria feel stigmatized from her association with Chernobyl and the charitable organization set up to support the children exposed to radiation? As a person with multiple chemical sensitivity, I knew the stigma of living with an environmental illness that others, including doctors, minimized or denied.

I couldn't know, nor could Maria, if she carried shame for a nuclear disaster that had occurred before her birth.

And, though Mike and I wouldn't refer to her as Indian, we would approach conversations with others about the girls with increased sensitivity.

Our vocabularies continued to expand in surprising ways.

One morning, the girls and I met a friend of mine in a quaint little town for a low-tide beach walk and lunch. Puget Sound displayed her jewels that day. Orange, red, and purple starfish clung to rocks. Sea anemones danced in tidal pools. Crabs skittered. Blue and purple mountains lay in the distance behind ferry boats riding the waves.

Intoxicated by the sea creatures and nature, we lost track of time until realizing we were ravenous. We hurried to a nearby café, a somewhat new experience for the girls. They'd never dined in a restaurant in Belarus, but they had already gone to a few with Mike and me. On each of those occasions they behaved well.

After the waitress took our order, the wait for our food seemed endless. Hungry and tired of waiting, Maria slumped in her chair, extended her long legs across the floor, and slammed her foot into Vika's. Vika howled and struck back, setting off a war of kicking and yelling.

"Stop!" I scolded. "No fighting!"

A few peaceful moments passed. Then Vika slipped under the table and barked like a dog, pawing Maria's legs like a puppy begging for food. This was not a new behavior. Vika loved dogs and loved pretending to be a dog. I found her antics amusing, at home, but now she was disturbing the peace in the restaurant and heads were turning our way.

For once, Maria ignored her. But Vika persisted. That's what puppies do.

Feeling like an inadequate mother, I pulled back the edge of the tablecloth and tapped Vika on the shoulder. She turned her head and gazed at me through thick bangs and soulful eyes.

"No, Vika. Restaurant. Sit in your seat," I said in a calm voice.

"*Woof!*" she barked at me.

Tired and starving, I wanted to growl back at her, but I felt the gaze of every person in the restaurant, waiting to see what I'd do next. So, I tried to channel Quan Yin, goddess of compassion and mercy.

"Lunch is coming soon. Sit in your chair," I said. My voice sounded far calmer and more patient than I felt.

Then Maria began to laugh uproariously, drawing even more attention to our table. I reached the end of my tolerance and raised my voice to Vika.

"Now!"

She crawled out from under the table. Poised on her hands and knees beside my chair, she looked up. "*Woof! Woof!*"

Convulsing with laughter, Maria rolled off the side of her chair and onto the floor. Now, I felt like one of *those* mothers, unable to control my children. My Quan Yin approach wasn't working. A different voice flew out of my mouth, unplanned.

"*Sidet seychas!*" *Sit now.* The words seemed to pop into my head from nowhere. Had I channeled the girls' mama? Their papa?

Shocked to hear those words come from me in their language, the girls shot into their seats and sat up straight, like magnets pulled to metal. I, too, was surprised by my ability to locate those two words, almost by osmosis, and by the power they wielded when spoken with a little oomph in the girls' native tongue. About the time the shock wore off, our food arrived, and they were again well-behaved little darlings.

Another day, we ventured out to play miniature golf. The first few holes induced big smiles, laughter, exclamations of excitement and disappointment. By the fifth hole, the girls were screaming for joy one minute, yelling at each other the next. On the sixth hole, Maria whacked the ball so hard it jumped over a barrier and disappeared.

"*Ahhhhhhhgh!*" She bellowed like a moose with its foot caught in a trap, then heaved her club through the air like a javelin and stomped off the course.

"Maria, where are you going?" Mike called. No answer. "Maria?"

"*Mashina!*" she retorted without stopping or turning around. *Car.*

"You can't go to the car by yourself," he hollered. Maria kept walking.

"You better go after her," I said.

Grumbling, he followed her. "I'll go to the car with you!" he yelled. When he caught up with her, he put his hand on her shoulder and tried to persuade her to finish playing the game. But Maria refused.

"We'll wait for you in the car," Mike informed me.

Vika's eyes met mine. "You want to play?" I asked, pointing to her ball.

"*Niet,*" she answered, her voice drenched in disappointment. On the drive home, Maria pouted in silence while Vika scolded her.

"Maybe she's homesick," I suggested to Mike.

"Yeah, maybe," he agreed.

At home, I roasted potatoes, steamed broccoli, and set the table while Mike grilled fish. As dinner cooked, I thought about how I might knit a reconnection with Maria and offer her a way back from where her outburst had flung her. Not wanting the golfing incident to color the mood at dinner, I went to find her.

As I stepped into the hallway, I saw Maria crouched in a lunge. With a grin on her face, she took a running start across the wood floor and slid right into me in her stockinged feet, arms open wide. *Bam!* Almost knocking me down, she planted a big, sloppy kiss on my lips. Without a word, we were reconciled. Falling in love with that volatile girl, I wrapped my arm around her, walked her to the kitchen, and handed her a bowl to carry to the table.

"Potatoes!" I announced.

"Kartoshka!" she responded.

"Fish!" said Mike, delivering a platter of grilled salmon.

"Ryba!" cried Vika, joining us.

"Ryba!" Mike and I repeated, adding yet another word to our growing vocabularies.

Before eating our dinner, we joined hands with the girls and, looking into their eyes, expressed our gratitude for their presence and the salmon on our table.

"I?" asked Maria, after Mike and I had spoken.

"Yes! Of course!" I responded, surprised by her desire to contribute to our ritual.

In a solemn tone, she spoke of her mama and papa, her sister, her *babushka*, Mike, and me. We understood that she was expressing gratitude for all of us. With each of her kin named, an image from the photo album the girls had shared with us came floating back to me. I felt a connection to an extended family, one I had yet to meet. Love wrapped itself around me like a warm summer breeze.

As we enjoyed our dinner, Russian and English words whooshed around the room like a flock of birds. When we finished eating, Mike slipped away from the table for a moment, then quick-stepped back with a bowl full of ice cream.

"Po Russkiy?" he asked. *How do you say this in Russian?*

"Marozhina!" the girls screamed with joy.

Little by little, with bits of English, Russian, hand signals, and mime, we were piecing together our own mother tongue. That night, as I tucked my twins into bed, I attempted to express my affection for them with a string of words in a new language.

"*Spokoynoy nochi, mynya krasivaya plavat ryba divchata.*"

Good night, my beautiful swimming fish girls.

CHAPTER 5

✳ It's All Relative

Humming with happiness, Maria and Vika swept the furniture and lamps with feather dusters while I put fresh sheets on the beds, plumped pillows, and assembled flower arrangements. Outside, a car slowed, pulled to the curb, and parked.

"They're here!" I called out. The twins came running to stand on the deck with me as Mike's sister, Debbie, and her three children poured out of their rental car and headed toward the stairs.

"You finally made it!" I hollered. It was their first visit to our Seattle home. With them living in Arizona, and us on the West Coast, our annual visits usually took place in Michigan when the clan gathered there for Christmas. They were making this summer trip for a family reunion that would bring relatives from the East Coast and Michigan to Seattle later in the week.

Deb's girl-next-door appearance hadn't changed. She was tall and slender with chin-length coffee-brown hair, fresh blonde highlights, and varnished fingernails. Over the years a comfortable closeness had grown between us, though she was more reserved and traditional than the women I tended to click with. Trooping up the stairs behind her—all sporting sunglasses, spanking-new Nike shoes, and head-phones plugged into their ears—the three kids grinned self-consciously. One by one, I wrapped them in hugs and introduced them to the twins.

"*Eto* Michelle," I said. "She's twelve." Michelle pulled out her earbuds and draped them over her shoulders.

"Hi," she said in a quiet voice. She was a shy girl with tight waves of golden-blonde hair framing her face.

"*Eto* Bobby. He's ten." Already aware of the power of his winning smile and wholesome face to attract girls, he continued to bob his head to music only he could hear.

"And *eto* Danny. He's seven." Danny, a skinny, long-legged kid with carrot-colored hair said hello and checked out Vika and Maria with a mischievous twinkle in his eyes.

"Show them in," I encouraged the twins with a sweep of my hand, hoping this would help to break the ice. They understood my request, happily shifted into roles as hosts, and led Debbie and the kids inside on a tour of the house.

I had hoped they would pause in the living room and dining area long enough for our guests to appreciate the best feature of our old fixer-upper—a broad view of the Olympic Mountains, with Puget Sound shimmering in the distance. Instead, they zoomed past the front windows and into the kitchen where they came to a halt in front of the dishwasher.

With our guests squeezed into a semicircle around them, Vika opened the door to the appliance as though unveiling a work of art. Maria demonstrated how to slide the racks in and out. An awkward pause followed as our guests waited for a revelation. My eyes darted around the circle. Debbie's smile had frozen in place. Michelle's eyebrows were scrunched together. The boys looked bored and confused. I could hear them all wondering: *Why are we looking at the inside of the dishwasher?*

In the tiny kitchens of Belarus and Ukraine, dishes were

hand-washed, then drip-dried on racks inside cupboards above the sink. At their *babushka's* house, I would learn, water for washing dishes had to be drawn from a well, carried home in buckets, and heated on the stove.

In the gated community where Deb and her children lived in Scottsdale, they were accustomed to homes with sprawling rooms, master suites, granite countertops and new appliances in the kitchens, and backyard swimming pools complete with water falling over rocks.

Now, standing in my kitchen, Maria and Vika appeared to be waiting for some indication that our guests understood we were living in the lap of luxury. They couldn't have known that dishwashers were as ubiquitous as denim jeans in the United States, or that our outdated model wasn't worth a dime.

"They're showing you the dishwasher so you'll know where to put your dishes when you finish eating," I explained to our guests. "They don't have dishwashers in Zalessie."

Michelle grasped the situation immediately. "Oh! Dishwasher!"

Satisfied, the girls smiled and headed toward the doorway leading to the back of the house. As the group followed them through the L-shaped kitchen, I cringed. The faded vinyl flooring needed to be replaced and the cupboard doors were overdue for a fresh coat of stain. But those were changes we couldn't make until safer, less toxic products came on the market. Even my 1950s stove, which I loved for its quirky, vintage charm, suddenly looked like a Goodwill donation. Standing next to the beautiful old crone—which I preferred over newer models—I began to feel self-conscious. What would Debbie and her kids think of a woman with no desire for the latest glass-topped model? After all, Americans are *supposed* to want the latest fashions, furnishings, cars, and gadgets to keep capitalism from skidding off the rails.

Though I liked creature comforts, I kept things for their aesthetics, practical value, and history, and I cared about the environmental impact of consumerism. Now, compelled by a blurry combination of shame and self-righteousness, I slapped my hand with a *thunk* on the shiny white enamel surface of my beloved stove.

"*This* baby is original to the house," I announced. "The Cadillac of stoves, high quality and built to last! They don't make stoves like this anymore—with chrome trim and all this workspace!"

"Does it work?" Danny asked, as though it might be a museum piece for display only. His red hair whorled at the crown.

"Oh yes!" I assured him. "Well, two burners work, anyway. The other two died, but the oven works fine!"

"Can't you get the burners fixed?" Bobby inquired, his skin tan and freckled by the Arizona sun.

"I had them fixed, once," I answered, slightly annoyed. "But they're on the blink again."

"Why don't you have it fixed again?" Bobby pushed. *When did he pull out his earbuds and start paying attention?*

"The repairman said he couldn't fix it again."

"Why not?" he pressed further. I was starting to feel hot and flushed. *You're a ten-year-old boy!* I wanted to say. *Why do you care?*

"The guy said something about a fire hazard," I mumbled, still trying to collect my thoughts. The moment that remark escaped my lips, I pictured our guests lying awake at night, terrified. I backpedaled. "Or it *could* be, I guess, if we're not careful. Really, the problem is, you can't get parts for these anymore. The less we mess around with it the better."

I glanced at Debbie. Her smile appeared to be painfully frozen. Her kids' faces told me they didn't understand my gushing. *They see a disaster waiting to happen.* The kitchen began to feel suffocating.

"Okay, let's move on, girls!" I said, pointing toward the doorway to the back hall. The group started to move, then Bobby paused his big feet in front of the refrigerator.

"Where's your ice dispenser?" he asked, dumbfounded. Everyone else stopped in their tracks and stared at the refrigerator.

"We don't have an ice dispenser. We use trays," I explained. Bobby's curiosity was grating on my nerves.

"Trays? What are trays?"

"You know, ice cube trays." I opened the freezer door beneath the refrigerator, slid out the bottom drawer, and grabbed a hot-pink plastic tray of ice. "Like this," I said, holding up the tray. "You just twist, like this," I explained, trying to rotate the ends of the slippery tray in opposite directions. "The cubes pop out," I went on, gritting my teeth and twisting harder. The ice wouldn't budge. My tingling cold hands twisted back and forth several times before those stubborn cubes loosened. One frozen block shot through the air, hit the ancient vinyl flooring, and disappeared under a counter. "See?" I said triumphantly.

"Oh yeah! My grandma used to have those at her house!" he remembered. Now I felt like a relic too.

"Keep going!" I encouraged the girls. While they moved on, I returned the tray to the freezer, threw the cannonball cube into the sink, and wiped my frosty hands on my jeans. When I rejoined them, the group had stopped again, just past the kitchen door. They were crowding into the pink-and-maroon tiled bathroom, a space smaller than Debbie's clothes closet. Wondering why on earth the girls had stopped in the bathroom, I prayed they wouldn't pull back the shower curtain to reveal the bathtub in all its chipped-and-stained-porcelain glory. My prayer was answered.

To my surprise and relief, the wall-mounted hair dryer was the showstopper. I wondered if a hair dryer was a luxury they didn't have at home, or if the attachment to the wall was what made it worth a stop on the tour. It didn't even occur to me that they might not have electricity, or their electrical power could be limited. I didn't consider that their mama and papa might view a hair dryer as an unnecessary waste of money, energy, and space. Maybe it's only in capitalistic countries, where "time is money," that people think they don't have time to let their hair dry naturally.

Maria removed the dryer from its cradle and switched on the blower. As it roared, I studied our reflections in the mirror above the vanity. Debbie's taut lips looked like a vise clamping two rows of pearly white teeth together. Open-mouthed, Bobby stared at Maria like a blind man whose sight had just been miraculously restored. A flicker of curiosity and wisdom registered in Michelle's eyes.

"Hair dryer!" she chirped.

"Nice," Bobby threw in, beginning to understand the complexities of cultural differences. Danny, smacking his gum, said nothing. We were all beginning to see the hair dryer from a new perspective. And I realized that through some people's eyes, our two-story house, filled with extra beds and linens and clothes and dishes, was a Taj Mahal. Our fifty-year-old pink-tiled bathroom with hot running water and fresh salt-air breezes floating in through the window was a Roman spa.

Certain that our guests had understood the hair dryer demonstration, Vika signaled Maria to wrap up the show. Maria expertly snapped the hot air wonder into its cradle and the blower stopped. Standing in the doorway behind the crowd, I backed out into the dark, narrow hall where we huddled elbow to elbow and elbow to wall. To escape the feeling of being trapped in a cave, I flipped on an overhead light. Its sudden brightness spilled into the doorways of two bedrooms and a small office. On the opposite wall was the door to the downstairs.

"*Eto* I and Maria," said Vika, standing at the threshold of the room the girls shared. Our guests peeked in to see a collection of stuffed animals on an old Mission-style bed, and a chiffonier inherited from my great-great-aunt Katie. A mirror affixed to Katie's dresser captured our images, beings from three different worlds.

"This one is mine and Mike's," I said, moving the group on to a slightly larger room furnished with a modern cherry sleigh bed, armoire, and nightstands. A jungle of Virginia creeper vines, visible through the open shades, ran amok on the back of the house and kept the room cool and comfortable.

For the first time, Danny spoke up. "Where's your TV?" he asked as though he'd never seen a bedroom with no television.

"Downstairs—where you're staying."

"You only have *one* television?" He sounded shocked.

"Yeah, we don't watch much television." I didn't mention to Danny that our television was a relic, not very big, and our basic cable service didn't include the twenty-four-hour sports channels he was used to. He would learn that soon enough.

"Let's go downstairs now," I continued, "right there behind you. Step aside so I can open the door!" An image of Debbie's spacious hallways flashed onto my mental screen as the kids backed into the bedrooms and bathroom to make room for the basement door to swing open.

Huddled in front of the dark, gaping hole of the stairwell, our pack of kids prepared to descend. "Careful!" I cautioned. "It's a little steep. Turn on the light so nobody falls!"

An invisible hand flipped the switch, illuminating the steps in multicolored rays of light shooting out of a disco ball hung on a chain from the ceiling. Red, yellow, blue, and green plastic gems covered the globe, except where a few had gone missing. Bright white light shone through those uncovered openings.

A silence fell over the group. No one moved or spoke for several seconds. When I could stand it no longer, I broke the trance.

"Take a look at that light!" I exclaimed, as though they hadn't already noticed. "You won't see that anywhere else, either!"

"Did you *buy* it?" Michelle asked.

"No, it came with the house. Probably original! I'm sure some collector would love to get their hands on it, but we're keeping it!"

"It's unique," Debbie commented.

"Okay! Let's go down. I'll show you where you're going to sleep."

The twins took the lead with the vigor of First Ladies showing guests to the Lincoln Bedroom in the White House. In the family room, the pullout sofa bed was layered in cotton sheets and blankets. Sunshine poured through the window blinds I'd made a point to open. Blue hydrangeas bloomed outside the window and draped their heads over a vase on a table beside the bed. On the floor were two mattresses I'd fashioned for the boys—cushions covered with bedding and pillows. The bulky old television sitting on a rolling cart at the foot of the bed drew no comments.

"Your little garden apartment is all set up!" I said, hoping our guests would find their daylight basement accommodations comfortable.

"Nice!" said Debbie, her smile now warm and authentic. She kicked off her shoes and relaxed on the sofa bed. I curled up in a chair.

At the other end of the room, Vika took a seat at the computer. Maria squeezed onto the chair with her. Ours was the first computer the girls had used. Both of them rapid learners, they could already play online games and search the internet for popular Russian musicians. It made no difference to them that it was not the fastest computer on the block.

Eager to flaunt her new skills, Vika clicked the mouse to open an app. With her shoulders pulled back and her face glowing with pride, she started a game. Soon Bobby gravitated to the girls.

"I can show you another game," Bobby offered after Vika's game ended. "You want me to show you?"

Tone and intuition translated his request in a way the girls understood immediately. They hopped out of the swivel chair so Bobby could sit. While he opened a different app and demonstrated how to play the new game, Vika watched dreamily and Maria clutched her throat and giggled. Before long, Danny joined them. The air was thick with hormones.

Something magical was happening in my Seattle home. An alchemy of cultures. Our niece and nephews and the twins were choosing to step toward, not away from, connection. Our differences had sparked a curiosity and attraction that was stitching us together with the beauty and warmth of great-great-aunt Katie's "crazy quilt"—a quilt traditionally made in North America of mismatched patches of varying sizes, shapes, colors, and fabrics handsewn together in a random pattern with an assortment of stitches from chevrons to chicken scratches.

Numbers of megabytes and television channels no longer mattered. The state of my linoleum became irrelevant. My house angst vanished. Deb and I exchanged smiles that said, *Yippee! The kids are bonding!*

CHAPTER 6

◈ Parenting 101

S inging a Russian pop tune on the front deck with Maria, Vika lifted a long-spouted watering can and sprinkled purple petunias and yellow daisies popping out of flower boxes.

I hated to interrupt their serenade, but we needed to get on the road to pick up Victor, the Children of Chernobyl chaperone, and show up on time for the girls' dental appointments.

"Time to go, girls!" I announced.

"One minute, Gail!" called Maria, her hair an uncombed mess.

"I go," said Vika. Wearing her favorite blue, green, and fuchsia spandex, she resembled a Picasso painting.

Under the circumstances, they seemed unusually calm and nonchalant. In Belarus, where teeth were repaired and removed without the use of anesthetics, dental care was avoided at all costs.

Victor had assured the twins this would be a "look and clean only" appointment. Still, I had expected them to be anxious and moody, if not belligerent, and I was glad he had agreed to accompany us.

Seated in the front seat with me, Victor chatted and bantered with Vika and Maria as we drove downtown. Not able to decipher more than a word here and there, I enjoyed the jazz-club ambiance of their repartee. Victor's deep baritone voice and the girls trilling high and low notes, punctuated with giggles and laughter, bounced off the car windows.

"... Mike ... *magazine ... dome* ..."

"... Mama *yi* Papa ... Babushka ..."

"... *plavat!* ... *Ozero* Washington ... Gail ..."

Hearing my name and Mike's in the exchange, I wondered if they were reporting to Victor their assessment of us. Their enthusiastic tone was reassuring.

Merging into a tangle of traffic, I exited the freeway in the heart of downtown Seattle and parked near the Cobb Building, a historic Fourth Avenue beauty trimmed with Native American sculptures and cornices. Once considered tall and glamorous, the eleven-story building had grown old and now was dwarfed by skyscrapers.

The girls raced through the quaint and quiet lobby to the push-button to call the elevator. Vika powered her way to first place.

"*Ya!*" she announced, pointing her finger to press the black disc. *I.*

A slow rumble sounded through the elevator shaft. A bell rang and the doors of the tiny elevator car opened at a slug's pace. We crowded in and I pointed to the button marked 11. Maria stabbed it with her index finger. After a pause, the doors closed and the compartment jerked to a start. Creaking and groaning, it carried us to our destination as though we had all the time in the world. At the eleventh floor there was a long pause, as if the old lift felt too tired from the climb to open her doors. When they finally parted, we entered a long, dimly lit corridor with white walls, closed doors down both sides, and a terrazzo floor. I worried the harsh cacophony of our footfalls would spook the girls. But it didn't seem to disturb them like it did me.

Must sound familiar to them, like stomping up the stairwell to their apartment in Zalessie, I surmised.

In a small office at the end of the hall, a receptionist greeted us warmly. Before we had time to take a seat in the waiting room, the hygienist arrived to usher Vika into a treatment room. Victor, Maria, and I trailed along behind and fanned out around the dreaded chair. Smiling nervously, Vika bravely took her seat on the mechanical throne. She hardly made a peep while the hygienist poked and cleaned and shined her teeth.

When the hygienist finished, in walked Dr. Turner, a quirkish man in his forties with a pointed chin. After a thorough examination of Vika's teeth, he announced they were "in good shape." Vika beamed. I breathed a sigh of relief.

"Give me five!" I said. Vika slapped my hand. Then it was Maria's turn to sit in the chair.

Anticipating she would receive the doctor's praises too, Maria scrambled into the seat. I sent up a silent prayer. *Please, God, don't let our luck run out.*

While the hygienist worked in Maria's mouth, Vika stood at the window, mesmerized by the view. Around us, a forest of high-rise office towers rose from the streets. Elliot Bay shimmered like a sea of jade and diamonds. The Olympic Mountains draped the horizon like a chain of amethysts. Ferries pulled in and out of the harbor.

We were sailing through the dental appointment on a warm, gentle breeze when Dr. Turner returned to examine Maria's teeth. Exuding the trust and confidence of an opera diva hitting a high note, Maria stretched her mouth wide open. The pink walls of her mouth and throat glistened under the beam of the doctor's tiny headlamp as he poked around with an instrument. After the examination, he put down his tool and pushed back his chair.

"She has three cavities that need to be filled." He spat

out the words like a radio announcer with breaking news of an imminent disaster. A shock wave rippled across the room.

By now the girls understood enough English to catch the drift of our conversation. Their internal radars screamed danger whenever the tone of a discussion regarding them implied anything unpleasant.

Maria's jaw clenched. Her face turned white. Vika whipped away from the window and stared at her sister, eyes opened wide.

"They will get worse and cause trouble," the doctor added. "You can set up an appointment at the front desk. We'll get her taken care of."

"Can you fill the cavities with a composite?" I asked. "I don't want you to use any mercury in her mouth. Her immune system is already challenged."

"That won't be a problem," he said, heading out the door to tend to his next patient.

Terrified, Maria shrank in the chair and faced Victor. "*Chto?*" she demanded to know. *What?* I was grateful it wasn't me who had to break the news.

"A little decay," Victor told her in Russian. "The dentist will take care of it, but not today." Maria grimaced.

"*Tri?*" she screeched. She had heard Dr. Turner say *three* and understood what that meant.

"*Da, tri,*" he confirmed. "But they are little. Don't worry. It's not like Belarus. Here you won't feel anything! Just a little pinch, that's all," he said in Russian. Most of the time Victor interacted with the children he chaperoned like a favorite uncle, but he was firm when necessary.

Maria's face turned sour, but she said nothing. She knew Victor expected her to be brave. Swallowing hard and pushing back tears, she tried. The last thing she wanted was for Victor to send her home early, a disgrace to her mama and papa.

"Home now," I said.

"*Davay*," said Victor. *Come on*. He tousled Maria's hair trying to console her, but she could barely shape her lips into a sad smile.

I scheduled an appointment for Maria for the following week, the only opening available before the girls returned to Belarus. With our time together running out, I hated to have our last ten days together end on a low note. But there didn't seem to be a better choice.

In the hallway, our footfalls echoed as we followed Victor and Maria to the car in silence. Vika leaned into me. Wondering what she was thinking, I slipped my arm around her. Was she relieved she had dodged a bullet? Experiencing survivor guilt? Feeling empathy for Maria?

Plenty of distractions in the days ahead prevented Maria from constantly stewing over the next appointment. Shopping for presents to take back to Mama, Papa, Elina, and Babushka. Swimming at the pool. A last trip to Seattle Center to ride the Ferris wheel and mechanical dinosaurs under the lights of the Space Needle.

Still, the reality of her upcoming appointment broke through between distractions. When the grim facts hit Maria, every drop of exuberance left her body. Her eyeballs sank into their sockets and her cheeks collapsed. Sometimes she pleaded, "I no dentist, Gail." Other times she expressed defiance. "I *no* dentist."

"It's going to be okay," I told her each time. "Not bad. You'll see." But nothing could soothe her. Then, like magic, a letter arrived from Zoya.

"*Pismo* from Mama!" I announced. The screen door slammed behind me. The timing of that letter couldn't have been more perfect.

The girls had begged me to let them have their ears pierced. I agreed to take them only with their mother's permission. Their telephone at home didn't receive long-distance calls, cell phones weren't in wide use in 1997, and social media didn't yet exist, so they had written her a letter. But the mail system was so unpredictable in Belarus that Vika and Maria had almost given up on receiving a response. It had been more than three weeks.

Now, giddy with excitement, they sat on the couch together and tore open the letter. Their eyes scanned each line of beautiful handwritten Cyrillic, in search of the answer to their question. Just before closing, Zoya had written "We give you our permission to have your ears pierced as long as Gail approves and does not find this to be an imposition."

Both girls jumped up from the couch and danced like jackpot winners in Las Vegas.

"Mama say yes! Mama say yes if Gail say okay!" Vika squealed, pulling on her earlobe in case I didn't understand.

I understood, and I joined them in happy dancing for a different reason. "Yaaay!" I cheered with them. "After Maria finish dentist, we go next day to get your ears pierced!"

Just as I'd hoped, Maria developed instant amnesia. There were no further protests against returning to the dentist. But a new wrinkle developed when Victor called to tell me that an unexpected situation had arisen that would prevent him from coming to the appointment with us.

"Don't worry, Maria will be fine," he tried to assure me. "She has already been there, already met the doctor. You will have no problem."

"I'm not so sure about that, Victor," I said nervously. "She's been very worried, and Maria can get pretty upset when she's scared." Victor hadn't seen her obstinate side, which, by now, I knew quite well. I remembered the scene at the miniature golf center, when she heaved her golf club into the air like a javelin and stormed off the course.

"I've explained everything to her, how it is here. She understands," Victor persisted.

I still wasn't convinced. Mike agreed to go with us, but even that didn't seem like enough support. I needed Ella.

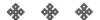

Ella, her husband, Alex, and their teenage daughter, Anna, were recent immigrants from Ukraine. Mike and I were introduced to them by a neighbor who worked in Anna's school when we were looking for Russian speakers who lived close by and could translate for us in a pinch after the twins arrived. We had hit it off immediately.

Hardworking and frugal, Alex and Ella had begun studying English the moment they landed in Seattle. As soon as they could understand and speak enough of the language to qualify for employment, Alex got a job moving furniture and Ella went to work in a delicatessen. By the time we met them, four years later, they had already bought a house, painted it pink, and rented out the upstairs to supplement their incomes. They were the kind of people who always said *Of course!* when others asked for help.

The twins loved spending time at their house, eating familiar foods and speaking in their native tongue. And they adored Anna, who watched them whenever I was busy meeting with psychotherapy clients.

"Of course, no problem," Ella reassured me now when I called to tell her about the current situation. "Vika can stay with Anna. I will go with you and Maria."

On "D" (dentist) Day, Maria's gaunt face, tight lips, and mournful eyes made me feel like a wicked witch sending her to six months of solitary confinement. When we arrived downtown and got out of the car, her long sun-browned legs didn't seem to know how to work properly.

"Come on, Maria," Ella said, placing a light hand on

Maria's back to help her gain momentum. "It is no big deal. I tell you the truth. I go to the dentist in this country many times."

With Ella's nudges, Maria's feet began to make progress.

Mike had arrived from his office ahead of us and now stood waiting in front of the Cobb Building. The historical structure that had, just one week earlier, looked to me like an elegant old lady, today appeared cold and masculine, like a prison. The lobby now struck me as dank and morbid, smelling of old colognes and cigarette smoke that had clung to the walls for decades.

When we approached the elevator, I waited for Maria to push the call button. But the thrill for her was gone. I pushed it myself as she stood staring at her feet, her head hanging low. A loud clunk announced the elevator's arrival. We waited for it to settle into place and watched the doors open in slow motion. On the eleventh floor, instead of a hallway lined with offices, I saw a tunnel of cells with locked doors.

Behind the door at the end of the hall, Dr. Turner and his assistant escorted us back to the treatment room. Maria sat in the chair like an inmate on death row. The doctor strapped on his surgical mask and tipped her chair back. His assistant handed him a syringe filled with lidocaine and fitted with a long needle. I cringed.

"Open wide, please," said Dr. Turner.

Maria gripped the arms of the chair. Her lips didn't move. Somehow the doctor slipped the needle into her gum.

"*Ahhhhhhhhhhhkkk!*" she screamed. And proceeded to gag.

Please let this be over soon, I prayed, certain that Maria would be fine as soon as the lidocaine numbed her mouth. But she continued to howl. My nervous system went ker-flooey when Dr. Turner fired up the drill and worked it into her mouth. Maria's wail matched the shrill whine of the machine. Every cell in my body screamed, *Get out of here!* But the mother's love and concern I felt kept me in the room. I would not abandon her. *She's not in pain, she's just scared*, I reminded myself. *All parents dislike this part of their job.* But the responsibility I felt for the well-being of another woman's child added to my burden, and my own fear escalated. *What if she has a rare complication and winds up in the hospital? What if she chokes to death on her own saliva? Thank God I'm not a full-time parent! Thinking about the potential threats to my children day and night would kill me!*

Dr. Turner struggled to keep the process going as Maria cried, snorted, and tried to turn her head away. "Wider, please," he gently requested over and over again. Each time Ella translated his request, her voice grew more sharp and stern.

I wanted to yell, *Stop*! But I knew it had to be done, so I held my tongue. *Better here, with sedation, than going to a dentist in Belarus to finish the job.* Mike's forehead furrowed and his jaw clenched as though he were anticipating a blow to his head. Even Ella grew weary and distraught. The yowl of the drill and Maria's terror wore on all of us.

Suddenly the drill went silent. The only sounds in the room now came from Maria. Whimpering. Coughing. Sucking air.

"I can't continue," said Dr. Turner. "I'm sorry."

Panic gripped me. "You can't stop now!" I gasped. "You've already drilled! She'll get a toothache or, even worse, an infection!"

"I can't do the work without a good line of sight, and the tooth needs to be kept dry for the composite to bond. We can't keep it dry or set the filling when she's this upset," the dentist explained, shaking his head.

"But what are we going to do? I can't send her home with a hole in her tooth! And what about the other two cavities? You said yourself, they'll only get worse."

"We can try again another day. Or you could take her to a pediatric dentist who uses nitrous oxide for sedation. That might work better for her."

Mike and I exchanged a look of shock. A pediatric dentist? Nitrous oxide? I didn't realize there were dentists who still used nitrous oxide, the "laughing gas" dentists used to sedate adult and child patients when we were children. Hadn't they all switched to newer drugs to block pain without the potential side effects of nitrous oxide? And who knew there were dentists who specialized in working with children? When we were kids, everyone in the family went to the same dentist. I cringed to think that we might have avoided this traumatic episode if Mike or I had known about this option. Guilt, shame, and regret seeped into my veins and turned my stomach. I had failed Maria. Failed parenting.

The Children of Chernobyl group was scheduled to return to Belarus in just a few days. It didn't seem possible to find a pediatric dentist who could finish the job on such short notice. The thought of needing to start over on another day seemed unbearable. I knew Maria would eat and breathe fear, day and night, until the next appointment. And there was no reason to believe the next appointment would be any easier.

Ella wasn't yet willing to give up. "You are a strong girl," she told Maria in Russian. "You need to cooperate. You don't want rotten teeth with terrible infection when you go home!"

"*Niet*, Ella," Maria sputtered. Weak, exhausted, and filled with shame, she closed her eyes. "*Niet.*" Her chin dropped and rested on her chest. I wanted to weep.

"It's pretty clear it isn't going to happen today," said Mike. "Let's go home. We'll figure it out later."

"If you find a pediatric dentist, I wish you well," said Dr. Turner as he rose from his chair. "Otherwise, give us a call and we can try again." He bid us goodbye and left the room.

His assistant removed the bib from Maria's chest and raised the back of her chair to an upright position. I picked up my shoulder bag and reached for the limp and lifeless hand of my beautiful swimming fish girl.

"*Davay*, let's go home," I said.

Like a mermaid on dry land, Maria hobbled out of the chair. Mike led us out the door.

"It's okay," I kept reassuring Maria as we walked to the rickety old elevator and rode down to street level.

Mike kissed me goodbye and headed back to work. "Try to relax now," he called over his shoulder. All of us were emotionally drained. Silent and pitiful, Maria crawled into the back seat of our Camry. Ella slipped into the passenger seat beside me.

"Maybe better to have Victor," Ella said mournfully. "Maybe Maria not so upset with him here."

"It's not your fault, Ella," I reassured her. "You did everything you could. It's my fault for not taking her to a pediatric dentist." The rest of the way, I drove in silence.

I parked the car in front of Ella's rosy-pink two-story house and turned to Maria. "Let's go in and get Vika."

"I car," Maria replied, her voice not much above a whisper.

"Okay. I'll be right back."

Inside, Vika and Anna were playing a game. When Ella and I walked in frazzled and without Maria, they were startled and confused. Wide-eyed, Vika turned to me.

"Where Maria?" She sounded alarmed.

"*Mashina*," I said. *Car.*

"What happened?" asked Ella's daughter.

Ella launched into a long explanation, in Russian. Shadows of worry darkened the girls' eyes as they absorbed the story. When Ella finished explaining, thirteen-year-old Anna glared at me in disbelief.

"She has to go back?" she yelped as though I were Cruella de Vil. I knew she already felt sorry for the girls for having to live with people who didn't speak their language. And it didn't help that every time the twins spent time at Ella's house, I had to pry them away when it was time to come home and they sulked all the way out the door. Of course, five minutes later, at home with Mike and me, they were happy campers again, but Anna didn't see that part of the picture.

"We're going to try to find a children's dentist where it won't be as scary," I explained in my calm mental-health-counselor voice. Inside I *felt* like Cruella and desperately wished I'd known about pediatric dentists before the debacle in Dr. Turner's office.

Champing at the bit to see Maria, Vika headed to the car without resistance, for once. I misinterpreted her eagerness, thinking she was worried about Maria and wanted to console her. Instead, she scolded and scowled.

What on earth is going on? I wondered. Then, Vika called to me from the back seat.

"Gail, ears tomorrow?" she casually inquired.

Now, I understood. She was concerned that, because Maria hadn't held up her end of the bargain, I wouldn't take them to have their ears pierced the next day.

I paused before answering her question. Part of me wanted to ask, *How in the world can Maria tolerate a needle through her earlobe but not a poke in her gum?* I knew I should stick to our deal and wait until after the completion of the dental work, but I decided there had been enough bad news and misery for one day.

"Yes, we'll get your ears pierced tomorrow," I said, certain I had just flunked Parenting 101. Again.

CHAPTER 7

◈ Baba Yaga

As we headed east on one of Lake Washington's floating
bridges, the North Cascade Mountains stretched out
across the horizon like a blue-hued watercolor of basalt and
granite. The twins, Victor, and I were on our way to a Seattle
suburb for Maria's appointment with a pediatric dentist. As
usual, Victor and the girls chatted in Russian.

"...Mama...Papa...," Vika trilled from the back seat.

The wind of change was picking up. In a few days, my
passengers would all fly away and disappear into a world
that was a mystery to me. I would remember this moment
as a dream.

"Papa . . . Moskva . . . ," Maria piped in. I gathered
she was relaying her papa's plan to meet their group in
Moscow to help transfer the kids and luggage to a bus for
their twelve-hour journey to Minsk, where the rest of the
parents would be waiting.

They're excited about seeing their mama and papa soon,
I mused. I pictured the girls, full of tales to tell, jumping from
the steps of the bus and landing on familiar ground. I imagined Zoya waiting with open arms, tears slipping from the
corners of her eyes. I hoped she and Ivan would be pleased
by how the trip had changed their girls. Never again would

their bewitching twins be dazed and frightened waifs setting foot on American soil for the first time. They were bilingual global travelers now, with experience of places their parents would most likely never see.

I'd been avoiding dwelling on it, but as the girls and Victor continued talking, my mind drifted to the coming separation. Thinking about our sometimes cozy, sometimes clamorous nest breaking up made me dizzy with a confusion of grief and exhaustion. The bonds we had created with the twins ran deep and strong. We were family now. How was I going to say goodbye to my girls, especially with no guarantee we would ever see them again?

At the same time, I knew I couldn't maintain the pace of a mother with twins much longer. My stamina had tanked. Umpteen appointments and outings with the girls, squeezed into seven weeks, had worn me out, partly from more chemical exposures than my normal life required. Barely holding on, I needed time for rest and self-care. Still, I couldn't imagine what life would be like with Vika and Maria no longer singing in the bathtub or dancing through the house.

"The girls want to know what kind of book you're writing," said Victor, interrupting my thoughts.

Surprised they had mentioned my book to Victor, it took a moment for his words to sink in. I planned to publish a book of narratives that would help others with environmental illness create meaningful lives and relationships despite the isolation and lack of medical support. I struggled to find the words to explain this to Victor.

"Well, I've been interviewing people from all over the United States and some from Canada who have an environmental illness called multiple chemical sensitivity," I began.

"Multiple chemical sensitivity?"

"Yes. It's also called MCS. People with this illness get sick from exposures to perfumes, scented laundry products, paint, glue . . . all kinds of ordinary products that are considered safe," I explained. "They have to isolate to avoid exposures. And they have to cope with the stigma of an illness many traditional Western doctors don't recognize." Wondering if Victor would think this was some strange American phobia, I took the risk of disclosing that I suffered with MCS myself. His response floored me.

"I have this too!"

"Really?" I was shocked. Like many people who are ill, including those with environmental illness, Victor appeared to be healthy.

"Yes! But in Belarus we don't have this name, multiple chemical sensitivity. We call it allergies." He seemed elated to discover someone who not only understood his bewildering experience but also had a name for it.

"All the time I ask my coworkers not to wear perfume," he continued. "Sometimes they forget, or they don't care and wear it anyway. My face turns bright red and feels like it is on fire, and it becomes difficult to breathe. I have to rush out of the room to recover. It is embarrassing!" His story tumbled out with the relief of finding he was not the only person suffering this way.

"I can't work in an office building," I confessed. "There are too many challenges for me. People wearing perfume or aftershave. Clothes laundered with scented detergent or dryer sheets. Cleaning products. Deodorizers and soaps in public restrooms. My brain gets jumbled. My ability to think is impaired, and I have trouble putting my thoughts into words. I have to meet with my clients in my home so the environment is safe for me."

"I can't be in the apartment when my wife uses laundry soap. It makes me very ill," Victor commiserated. "I tell her to wear a mask when she washes our clothes and cleans the house because I don't want her to get sick too."

"We clean our house with vinegar and baking soda," I said. "That works for just about everything. We wash our clothes with unscented laundry detergent, use baking soda instead of fabric softeners, and never use dryer sheets—those are really toxic."

"I can ride the bus in Minsk until it gets crowded. Then I have to get off and walk the rest of the way because I feel like I am dying. My son gets very ill from car exhaust." Victor spoke slowly and his words carried a tone of sadness. "He avoids taking car trips because he feels so terrible and embarrassed by this condition."

"Car exhaust makes me sick too. Whenever I'm in the car, I keep the exhaust fumes out by keeping the air vents and windows closed," I told him.

"Ahhh," Victor said, nodding. I could almost see the wheels turning inside his head, thinking how this strategy might help his boy. After swapping stories and coping strategies, we touched on the roots of the illness.

"In the US, the air, food, and water are full of pesticides and other neurotoxins and hormone disruptors that damage the immune system and impair brain development in children."

Victor chuckled ruefully. "Fortunately, in Belarus there is no money for pesticides."

"Radiation harms the immune system too. I wonder if the radiation from Chernobyl makes you more susceptible to low-level chemical exposures."

"I don't know. I've wondered about that too."

The girls giggled and prattled in the back seat, expressing no interest at all in the conversation taking place up front. Unbeknownst to the twins, they had created an important connection between Victor and me. Our talk now turned to the devastating effects of invisible pollutants, denied by our cultures and difficult to prove or measure.

"Hanford is another example," I said. "It's a former nuclear weapons plutonium plant in Eastern Washington that's been shut down for many years, but radioactive contaminants are still leaking into the soil and groundwater."

"Yes, I've heard of Hanford."

"Hanford employees and downwinders were used in nuclear experiments without their knowledge. People who suffered from cancer and other debilitating health conditions related to radiation exposure were ignored for decades. The nuclear cooling systems contaminated the Columbia River. And spills weren't always accurately reported. The whistleblowers—employees who complained about safety issues at the plant—lost their jobs."

Victor sighed. "I remember the day I learned we were in danger from radiation in Belarus. The Soviets hadn't yet announced the accident at Chernobyl. I received a phone call from a friend. He said, 'Something has happened. There's been a big spike in radiation. I've seen the readings. I don't know the source, but something's going on. Something terrible.' I understood immediately, this was not a warning to ignore."

"What did you do?" I asked.

"I slammed down the phone and rushed out the door. My son was visiting his grandmother in the countryside. I knew he would be playing outdoors, the worst place he could be if radiation levels were high. I drove into the wind for two hours to get there. My heart was racing all the way. And I kept hoping maybe it was an error in the reading, a false alarm." Victor paused. Grief saddened his eyes.

"If they had warned us about the radiation," he continued, "we could have taken iodine. Everyone in Belarus has it in their medicine cabinet. Iodine will block radiation from damaging the thyroid. It would have been so simple. But we didn't know." A quiet fell over us.

When we arrived at our destination, a modern, low-rise office building, the twins stopped talking too. Their silence gave me pause. *What if Maria can't do this?* My stomach tightened. I turned off the ignition. Victor's focus had shifted too. Now, his eyes twinkled with mischief.

In a slow, easy voice that carried a hint of intrigue, Victor turned and spoke to Maria. Something about Baba Yaga and *marozhina*. His head looped from side to side as though his neck had lost control. The girls fell into fits of laughter. Maria emerged from the car, calm and good humored.

"What in the world did you say?" I asked.

"I told Maria this doctor she will see today is a Baba Yaga with magical powers. This Slavic witch will make Maria feel very happy, like she is drunk. But not drunk on beer, drunk on ice cream!"

As we entered the building, a waft of fragrance drifted our way from a cluster of people waiting for the elevator. Knowing perfume could make me sick, Maria looked at me and pinched her nose as a warning, in case I hadn't yet detected the smell. She and Vika were used to my condition and helped me to avoid exposures when they could. Now I was grateful that Victor understood too. Without a word spoken, none of us made a move to step into the elevator with the scented women. Instead, we waited for the next one.

The sleek elevator quietly swooshed us to the third floor. The doors opened without delay. We stepped into a wide, carpeted corridor where modern art hung on the walls. The surroundings oozed with the warmth and luxury of a resort. As we entered the dental office, we passed a smiling child on his way out. There were children's books scattered on tables and a play area filled with toys. I gave Maria the thumbs-up sign, code for, *This place is awesome!* She smiled and took a deep breath.

The three of us were ushered into a room with a child-sized dental chair that looked like a cozy La-Z-Boy recliner. The dentist, a middle-aged Eastern European woman with dark hair and olive skin, took Maria under her wing.

"Seet right here and get com-fort-a-ble," she instructed Maria in a hypnotic voice. "I will lay you back so you can relax, and I'll put this little oxygen tube right by your nose so you can breathe very well. It will make you happy!"

The oxygen mixed with nitrous oxide calmed Maria instantly. She rested like a baby suckling milk while the doctor took care of her three cavities.

"Finished!" Maria cheered when we walked out the door. Baba Yaga had not let us down.

Part Three:

1998

CHAPTER 8

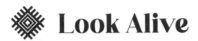 **Look Alive**

The Children of Chernobyl organization based in Minsk survived another year, despite threats from the government to discontinue the practice of connecting Belarusian and Ukrainian children with the Western world. After an eighteen-hour delay in their flight from Moscow, due to a mechanical problem, Maria and Vika returned for their second visit to Seattle on the Fourth of July 1998, which also happened to be my forty-sixth birthday.

When my alarm sounded at 3:00 a.m., I hurried into my clothes. With little sleep, Mike and I set out for the airport, in the dark, for their 5:00 a.m. arrival. Still groggy, Mike said almost nothing as he drove. I, on the other hand, couldn't keep quiet.

"Do you think they'll feel shy at first, after not seeing us for so long?" I chattered.

"I wonder how they will have changed," I pondered.

"Maybe they'll feel right at home."

I couldn't wait to tell the twins I had enrolled them in a swimming class, *and* the four of us would be taking a trip to Lake Chelan, a popular vacation spot in Eastern Washington.

As passengers funneled into customs, I scanned their faces, searching for Vika's charming puppy smile and Maria's

irresistable grin. Suddenly I caught fragments of familiarity—
the turn of a head, a profile that made my heart leap.

"There's Vika! She's in the lavender sweatshirt and red
pants."

"I see her!" Mike confirmed, excitement mounting in his
voice. "And there's Maria right behind her!" At that same
moment, Maria spotted us. She smiled impishly and tossed
her arms in the air.

When they came through the glass doors, we four melted
into a huddle and my concerns vaporized. This was a family
reunion. Carrying the fragrance of crackers and peanuts,
the twins were now experienced travelers, returning to their
second home. Their honey-colored hair bobbed at their
shoulders. Both girls had grown taller, but Vika had not yet
caught up with Maria.

"I'm so glad you're finally here!" I said, my eyes brimming
with tears.

Mike opened a bag, pulled out two Disney T-shirts—one
purple and one pink—and held them up. Maria chose the
purple one. "Mickey Mouse! *Spacibo!*" Her knobby knees
would poke out beneath that T-shirt all summer.

"Tigger!" Vika cheeped. *"Spacibo!"*

We collected their bag from the carousel—the same small
black duffel they had arrived with the previous summer—and
headed home. This time, the girls scrambled into the car and
buckled themselves in. Instead of uncomfortable silence, our
wide-eyed girls, now nine years old, pointed to landmarks
they remembered as we drove over the old Seattle viaduct.

"Ferry boat!" Vika cried.

"Space Needle!" Maria exclaimed, pointing toward
Seattle's signature landmark at the foot of Queen Anne Hill.

"Fish park!" they squealed in unison, remembering the
parade of boats, jumping salmon, and fish ladders as we
drove past the Ballard Locks.

When we arrived home, they rushed out of the car and raced to the house. With necks extended and noses pointed, they paused just inside the door, sniffing for familiar scents, then rushed to "their" room. On the bed lay Tweety Bird backpacks we'd bought for them. Bursting with happiness, I wanted to turn cartwheels while they puzzled out the trick of strapping on the packs.

After mastering the backpacks, Vika lunged for the bag they'd brought from Zalessie and pulled on its cranky old zipper in fits and starts. Impatient, Maria tried to squeeze her hand through a tiny opening.

"*Niet!*" Vika growled.

Here we go, off to the fights! I thought. But, to my surprise, Maria backed off. I hoped this was a new level of self-restraint and maturity, an indicator there would be less fighting between the girls this summer. When the bulging duffel released its grip on the overflowing treasure trove of gifts, both girls plunged their hands inside.

"Gail, for *happybirthday!*" said Vika, presenting me with a wristwatch. The twins always said *happybirthday* as if it were one word, as in, when is your *happybirthday*? I slipped the silver-toned watch over my wrist.

"You remembered my birthday? *Spacibo!*" I gushed. Vika's eyes twinkled.

"Gail, Babushka make!" Maria proudly explained as she draped a cross-stitched table runner across my lap.

"*Krasivaya!*" I exclaimed, picturing her grandmother working a needle and colorful threads on dark winter nights when snow covered the roof of her cold, drafty house in a tiny Ukrainian village. *Beautiful!*

When the gift-giving ritual ended, we teamed up to prepare breakfast. Mike cooked sausage, I fried potatoes and eggs, Vika poured milk, and Maria set the table.

"We sleep Cosmos!" Maria exclaimed as we worked together, referring to one of Moscow's most elite hotels. When their flight was postponed, the airline had provided the group with overnight accommodations at the Cosmos.

"Yes! I heard! That must have been exciting!"

"*Ya yi* Maria one!" Vika added.

"Oh! You and Maria had your own room?" I said, feeling in sync with the twins. Without missing a beat, we were speaking in the mother tongue we'd pieced together the previous summer.

"*Da!*" they sang in unison.

"One girl no good morning," said Maria, pretending to slit her throat with her index finger. Her head dropped to the side. Eyes rolled skyward. Her tongue dangled from her mouth.

Though anyone else might have deduced that one of the children had croaked in her room at the Cosmos, I knew this was Maria's way to communicate endings of many kinds. But I couldn't imagine what on earth had happened at the hotel.

"Victor break door! '*Samolet, dyesat minuty!*'" Vika added, mimicking Victor's gruff voice. *Airplane, ten minutes.*

"Was the girl okay?" I asked, befuddled.

"*Da.* She sleep." Now it all made sense.

"She didn't hear her alarm and overslept?"

"*Da!*"

"Victor had to pound on her door to wake her up, ten minutes before you had to leave for the airport?"

"*Da! Da!*"

With breakfast on the table, we took our seats and joined hands. Before I said a word, Maria jumped in.

"I, *pozhaluysta?*" *Please.*

"Yes!" I said, thrilled she wanted to say a blessing.

"*Spacibo* Mama *yi* Papa . . . Gail," she said, sitting tall. "Michael," she continued, turning her eyes to him. "Elina *yi* Babushka . . ." When she finished, three generations of her family and ours had been blessed by a young girl who wanted us to see how much she had matured since her previous visit. I was touched by seeing the beauty of ritual awakened in her. Of course, it wouldn't be long before we'd realize her wild streak trailed not far behind.

After filling their tummies, Maria and Vika ran out of steam.

"Time for a bath!" I announced. "If you get some sleep this afternoon, we'll go watch the fireworks on Lake Union tonight! *Boom! Boom!*" I used my arms and hands to indicate fireworks exploding.

Squealing with delight, the twins scurried to the bathroom and began filling the tub. Just as they finished bathing and were about to nap, the telephone rang.

"This is Dan from *KING 5 News*," said the caller. "I understand you and your husband are hosting a couple of kids from the Children of Chernobyl group. We'd like to come out and interview you and the children for tonight's evening news."

Momentarily stunned, I paused, searching for words. The last thing I had expected was to make a television appearance. The idea made me nervous. I was accustomed to talking to groups in my role as a mental health counselor, but television—without a script—required a step way beyond my comfort zone. Yet this was an opportunity I couldn't pass up, an opportunity to increase awareness of environmental dangers in our own country as well as Belarus. An offer that I knew might never come my way again.

The twins had been in the house for less than two hours and were already attracting people and opportunities like a pair of lucky dice. Once again, they had unwittingly acted as conduits for an environmental information highway, the way they had the previous summer when they prompted

Victor to ask about the book I was writing and I had learned of his struggle with MCS.

"Uh, oh-kay," I replied, trying to wrap my brain around the idea.

"Do you have any plans to celebrate the Fourth?" Dan asked, searching for an angle.

Though it was a perfectly natural and harmless question, it irked me. In my mind, Dan wanted to spin a patriotic "Land of the Free, Home of the Brave" kind of story. *He wants to set Mike and me up to play heroes*, I thought, picturing Mike wearing a ten-gallon white hat and dusty cowboy boots. *Then, he'll cast the girls as cute, eager recipients of US charity and unwitting converts to democracy. What if he reinforces the polarization of our two countries?* My inner voice ranted on and on. *He'll yak on and on about the Soviet cover-up of the Chernobyl disaster and ignore the government-sanctioned environmental disasters in the US, including radioactive pollutants!*

I took a deep, calming breath before speaking. "Well, we *might* go to the fireworks," I said hesitantly. My palms were sweating. I glanced up. Vika and Maria stood nearby, listening. Seeing their faces bright with innocence and curiosity gave me the courage to suggest a different angle. I took a breath. "There's something else I'd like to talk about."

"What's that?" Dan asked.

"Well," I gulped, "I'd like to talk about environmental issues—in Belarus *and* here, in the US," I began. "My husband and I volunteer as host parents for the Children of Chernobyl group because we know from personal experience how devastating toxins in the environment can be. The girls' immune systems are compromised from exposure to radiation, making them more vulnerable, and I have an illness called MCS—multiple chemical sensitivity." Fearing Dan would decide not to interview us after all, I braced myself for his response.

"We're on our way!" Dan's sudden burst of enthusiasm startled me.

Oh no! What have I gotten us into? Before I could consider backing out, the deal was done.

"We'll be there in twenty minutes," Dan informed me with the urgency of a newsman chasing a breaking story. Shocked and excited, I hung up the phone.

"Ohmigod!" A shot of energy ping-ponged up and down my spine. Part of me felt thrilled, another part feared stepping into the spotlight, speaking about an important but controversial subject. *Am I setting myself up to be judged or ridiculed?* For several seconds I stood frozen, my mind racing, until Vika broke my trance.

"What, Gail? *Chto?*" she demanded. Her question brought me back to earth like a spent Roman candle. My resolve quickened. It was Independence Day, *and* it was my forty-sixth birthday. Time to exercise my freedom! I had a right to tell the world—on television—that environmental illness, caused by nuclear disaster or by chemical pollutants, was real and global. I had a duty to warn Americans of the dangerous trade secret cover-ups lurking in our cupboards.

"You, Maria, Mike, and I talk on television!" Vika gawked at me.

"We? Television?" With their eyebrows knitted in confusion, Vika and Maria exchanged glances, still disbelieving.

"I'll call Ella. She'll explain in Russian," I said, already punching her number into the phone. While the girls talked to her, I poked my head into the bedroom where Mike was napping.

"Look alive!" I cried. "*KING 5* is coming to interview us!"

"What?" Confused and groggy, Mike rubbed his eyes.

"*KING 5 TV News!* Here in twenty minutes! Look alive!"

I sped around the house clearing dishes from the table like a woman with her hair on fire and tried to quiet my monkey brain. *Thank God no one watches the five o'clock news on the Fourth of July!* At the same time, another inner voice proclaimed, *It's my responsibility to speak the truth!*

Vika had stationed herself in the front window with binoculars. "*Mashina!*" she yelled when the KING 5 truck pulled up and parked across the street. Through the binoculars, she watched two men emerge from the vehicle. One carried a large camera on his shoulder. Though she didn't realize it, her TV debut had already started—the cameraman was filming her through the window.

When Vika announced the crew's arrival, Maria bolted like Paul Revere to alert Mike and me, in case we hadn't heard. "Gail! Mike! *Mashina!*" Rushing helter-skelter, the three of us almost collided in the hallway.

A second wind had struck the girls. Wide awake now, they vibrated with adrenaline, though the moment the newsmen walked through the door, both girls clammed up. Dan took a seat, while the other man stood working the camera. When Mike and I sat, the girls climbed onto our laps like curious cats.

"Has Maria's or Vika's health been impacted by radiation?" Dan inquired.

"Their immune systems are compromised, and they are at risk for developing serious health issues, including thyroid cancer," I explained. "All of the children who come are screened for cancer by a University of Washington clinic."

"Maria already has digestive problems," Mike added.

"I'll bet you wish they could stay here, where they wouldn't be exposed to radiation," said Dan, his eyes locked on mine. This was the opening I had hoped for. My chance.

"In some ways, yes," I agreed, swallowing hard. "But here in the US, children are developing chronic illnesses from chemicals in *our* air, food, and water. Pesticides used in their homes, their schools, and on their playgrounds contain carcinogens and neurotoxic chemicals that impair their immune systems and brain development."

I wanted to remind viewers of the US government's own history of nuclear radiation cover-ups. But I knew I'd be more effective if I kept my message short and sweet. "We need to protect *all* of our children," I said emphatically.

"You mentioned you have an environmental illness," Dan commented.

"Yes, I have MCS—multiple chemical sensitivity," I said. "I get sick from exposures to ordinary products most people assume are safe." Wishing I had an easy explanation, I turned to Mike. He immediately jumped in for me.

"You wouldn't intentionally ingest poison, right, Dan? But that's what happens when you plug in a room deodorizer, or use cologne, or wash your clothes with scented detergents or dryer sheets," he said.

I could feel Maria beginning to get restless and impatient. Then, she jabbed her foot into Vika's leg. Vika jabbed back. A full-blown battle was brewing with the camera rolling.

"*Niet!*" I whispered to Maria. She moved her feet back to where they belonged. Vika smirked. I raised my eyebrows as a warning to her.

Dan segued to a different topic. "How do you communicate with these girls? Do you speak Russian?"

"They teach us Russian words and they've learned some English. We mix it all up, and it seems to work!" I explained.

"What activities do you enjoy together?"

"We like to play UNO in two languages," Mike answered.

"Show us how you play UNO!" suggested Dan.

Now we were talking the twins' language! Without a word, Vika popped off Mike's lap, opened a drawer, and pulled out the cards. Mike and I followed the girls to the dining table. Maria shuffled and dealt like a pro as the camera rolled.

"*Zheltyy!*" we all yelled when Maria turned over a card.

"*Po* English?" Mike asked.

"Yellow!" the girls called out. Naming each color in two languages, we showed television viewers how easily people without a shared language could enjoy playing a game together.

Vika was first to cry "UNO!" On the next round, she turned over her last card. "Zero!" she exclaimed, using the word that, in our vocabulary, meant *finished*.

"*Niet!*" Maria protested. Slumping in her chair like an empty flour sack, she closed her eyes, and, using her index finger as a butcher knife, pretended to slit her own throat. "*Kkkhhhaaaahkkk.*" The sound effect was dramatic. In a single movement, her chin swung to the side and dropped to her shoulder, her tongue protruded from her mouth and dangled. Spittle appeared on her lips. Captured on camera, this went down as one of Maria's finest performances.

After the reporter and cameraman left and our adrenaline settled, the girls napped. When the news hour approached, we gathered around the television in the basement, all of us giddy with excitement and fatigue.

"There's Vika!" exclaimed Mike when the screen came to life.

The twins hooted and laughed as we watched Vika on-screen, cute as a button, gazing out the window through binoculars that were way too large for her face. The image was sure to capture viewers' attention. But something about it made me uncomfortable. Was it intended to portray her as a little Russian spy? I bristled at the idea of projecting a Russian stereotype onto a young child, however innocently.

As Vika "spied," an off-camera anchorman delivered a teaser. "A group of children escaping radiation from Chernobyl arrived in Seattle today from Moscow. Could *your* children be at risk *too*? Coming up next on the news at 5."

His deep voice sounded ominous. The station cut to a commercial break.

After the break, the anchorman announced that local volunteers for an international humanitarian aid group were hosting the radiation-exposed children. "Here's Dan with that story."

The scene shifted to Mike and me in our living room with the twins sitting quietly on our laps. "The food, fresh air, and vitamins they get here boost their immune systems," Mike explained to Dan. The camera zoomed in on Maria, all skin and bones, her hair tousled. Then the camera turned to me.

"We need to protect *all* of our children from environmental toxins," I added. Taken out of context and stripped of relevance, my statement fell flat. On that note, the clip ended and the anchorman reappeared to wrap up the story with a final comment.

"This local couple is concerned that chemicals in our own environment could harm children too. Up next, we'll tell you about the weather you can expect for tonight's fireworks. Stay tuned."

My heart sank. Our moment of fame had lasted less than thirty seconds, a collection of shallow sound bites that overlooked critical issues and did nothing to educate the public about serious threats to their own health. That story had been cut along with Maria's dramatic performance.

"That's it?" I asked.

"That's it," Mike answered matter-of-factly.

The girls were exuberant. "I say Mama, Mama say 'no!'" exclaimed Vika.

"Your mama won't believe it when you tell her we were on television?"

"*Da!*"

The girls' joy pushed my disappointment aside to create space for a different perspective, one related to the way images traverse the heart and soul in regions where no words exist. Curiosity bubbled up in me. What if the story that aired would be more potent *because* of its fluff? Our television appearance, I realized, had shown viewers a powerful image of ordinary people choosing to create connection and love despite barriers of stereotypes, politics, and language. Wasn't that the choice our nations needed to make in order to heal our complex environmental, social, and political issues? I hoped that the image of our family launching into our second summer together told a more important story than I could have spoken.

Soon we were off to join the crowd of people gathered near Lake Union for the fireworks. On the lake, boats formed an arc around a barge where pyrotechnicians prepared a spectacle of explosions. When darkness fell, the show began. *Kaboom! Kaboom! Kaboom!* Fiery patterns splashed across the sky—flowers, stars, and waterfalls expanding and floating toward us like deities about to swallow us whole. Rivers of light popped and danced and flowed from the sky, illuminating every face with awe. In that sea of faces, I saw untold stories of freedoms lost and found. We were all swimming in rivers of joy and sorrow.

CHAPTER 9

❖ Learning to Swim

Yipping and splashing, fifteen little swimmers clung to the side of the pool waiting for class to begin. The instructor, a boy sporting mirrored sunglasses and a perfect tan, perched on the lifeguard tower. With legs spread wide, knees pointed at opposite ends of the pool, he lifted a megaphone to his lips with one hand.

"Number off!" he yelled like a drill sergeant. "*One-twothreefour!* When your number is called, swim across the pool and wait. Don't go until your number is called!" He didn't appear to be old enough to own a driver's license.

As the wiggly kids began to number off, my mama reflex struck me with an intense urge to run over to Vika to make sure she understood the instructions. Another inner voice suggested I sit back and wait. *Don't be a helicopter parent.* She showed no signs of distress as she watched and listened to the kids around her with rapt attention. *She doesn't need to be rescued.* I leaned back on the chaise lounge and listened to numbers slapping the air.

Vika called out her number correctly when it was her turn. *That's my girl!* I thought. The moment the last kid called out his number, the instructor's voice blasted through the megaphone again.

"*Threeone!*"

My spine tightened a notch when he called out two numbers as though they were one. With a nervous smile painted on her lips, Vika watched half the kids push off the wall. I saw confusion on her face, wondering whether she, too, should have launched. My mama bear voice growled in my head. *Geez! Would it have killed you to call out just one number at a time? Maybe talk a little slower?* I had explained to him, right before the class had begun that morning, that Vika didn't speak much English but would understand him if he spoke to her directly and not too fast. Now it seemed like he might be purposely trying to confuse her.

Before the ones and threes reached the other side, Mr. Megaphone yelled again. "*Fourtwo!*"

The remainder of the swimmers shoved off. Not about to be left behind, Vika plunged in after them. While she made her way across the water, I stationed myself poolside to meet her.

"Good job!" I said, squatting beside her. Wearing lime green goggles, she beamed with pride.

I rose and stood where the instructor couldn't miss seeing me, hoping he would recall our earlier conversation if I made myself more visible. I could have sworn he was looking directly at me with a twisted smirk on his face. My eyes pleaded with him. A knot formed in my stomach and I felt dizzy from the chlorine fumes rising from the pool.

"Sound off! *Elephantgiraffetigerhippopotamus!*"

A bolt of anger shot through me. I clamped my hands on my hips. There was no doubt in my mind that he made himself feel more high and mighty by making the class more confusing for Vika. I wanted to knock down his tower as he leaned back with the self-importance of power. Then the firing of my maternal synapses redirected me to Vika.

"You giraffe," I said, squatting beside her again. "When teacher says 'giraffe,' you go!" Squinting with one eye, she looked up at me and nodded, her face lit with joy. If the instructor was giving her a hard time, she didn't know and didn't care.

Less quick but more graceful than any of the others, she set off when the giraffes and hippos were called. While the tigers and elephants took their turns, I walked to the deep end of the pool to check on Maria's class. Sheer stamina had landed her in the more advanced class, though her technique reminded me of a cat skating on ice. Her arms and legs flailed every which way, splashing water. Her instructor, a young woman, stood on the pool deck and made eye contact with all of her students, including Maria. Speaking in a calm voice, she made certain that everyone understood the instructions, and she offered tips and encouragement. *Now that's the way to teach a class! Inclusive communication! Clarity! Positive feedback! Mr. Megaphone could learn a thing or two from her!*

Knowing Maria was in good hands, I circled back to Vika's end of the pool. Her instructor continued to issue confusing orders from his aerie as though the distance between him and the swimmers afforded him an extra dose of authority. A fire roared in my belly. My inner voice raged. *That boy shouldn't be allowed to work with children! Someone needs to teach that brat a lesson. I don't care that he's young and inexperienced, he works for the City of Seattle and he should know better!*

This boy had ignited in me the memory of another incident, when I had been targeted by a bully, a woman who also happened to work for the City of Seattle, in a management position. She and I had both enrolled in a class for people interested in discussing the art and joy of living more simple, less-materialistic lives.

My sensitivity to fragrances was so severe at that time that I was not able to attend many group events without becoming ill. I had decided to take that risk because it seemed to me that if anyone would understand and respect my need to avoid toxic exposures it would be people who were interested in healthier, more simple lives. I took the chance and signed up, knowing that if it didn't work out, I could drop out. The first meeting heartened me. Six of us sat around an old wooden table and there were no offending scents. When asked to introduce myself, I mentioned my chemical sensitivity and explained it would be helpful to me if my classmates refrained from wearing fragrances. Everyone had seemed amenable. All went well until the final meeting of the class.

When I arrived that evening, I took a seat and chatted with classmates, as always, while waiting for the instructor and other students to arrive. I had no clue that one of the participants we were waiting for was an assailant who had intentionally doused herself in strong perfume in order to attack me that night.

Instead of taking her usual place at the opposite end of the table, the woman walked in and squeezed in beside me. Her perfume hit me with chemically induced brain fog. Though I knew I needed to leave the room immediately, my impaired brain scrambled my ability to respond.

Dazed, I turned to the woman and asked, "Are you wearing perfume?" It was a ridiculous question to ask, but my thoughts were tangled. I couldn't compute that a grown woman, one who worked in a leadership position, would intentionally try to harm me.

"Yes!" she snarled. "To prove that your chemical sensitivity is bullshit! I've worn perfume to every class and it never bothered you before!" The hostility in her voice was cold and vile. Stunned, I couldn't imagine why my health problem had angered her, why she would turn herself into a chemical weapon to harm me.

One part of my brain kept telling me, *Leave the room! Now! You need to get out!* But a disconnect between my

head and my limbs immobilized me. Revved up and mis-
firing, my brain cells were stuck in neutral like a race car
unable to cross the starting line. Finally, I willed myself to
stand up and walk out. Dizzy and confused, I stumbled to
my car and sat there until my brain cleared enough for me
to drive.

Now, at the pool, watching a young American man
wielding his morsel of power, all I could see was a bully.
Though he had not plotted an attack, as had the woman in
my class, he had ignored my request for him to put just a
little effort into helping Vika understand the instructions.
In fact, he seemed to make the instructions as confusing as
possible. That, combined with off-putting body language
and a simpering smile, struck me as a form of abuse, a form
too subtle to prove. That perception wound me so tight with
anger that the story in my head allowed no room for any
other perspective. It would be years before I would consider
the possibility that his behaviors were unconscious or not
mean-spirited.

As a professional counselor, I knew how to work with
bullies. But, at the pool, my role as a protective mother
took precedence. My therapeutic techniques flew away like
a flock of starlings. I was a grizzly mama bear protecting
my baby. I didn't want to approach this boy respectfully. I
wanted to knock him off his chair and push him underwater.

Lost in my fantasies of vengeance, suddenly I noticed
Vika waving to me, dripping with pleasure and glory. Her
concave spine, pushed-out chest, and open-mouthed smile
screamed, *Look at me! Look at me!*

I took a long, deep, calming breath. Vika's innocence,
I realized, provided all the protection she needed in that
class. She had expected to be lost due to the language barrier and wouldn't let that stop her. In fact, she may have
found the instructor's authoritarian demeanor familiar and

comfortable, challenging in a positive way. And, she had figured out that it didn't matter which group she belonged to when the teacher mixed things up every two minutes. She jumped in wherever she wanted to, thrilled to be learning to swim. Not wanting to do anything to burst that bubble, or draw unwanted attention to her, I realized the best course of action was for me to do nothing.

Though I still disliked the instructor's alpha style, I felt a weight lift from my chest. Now, the din of children jabbering, teachers yelling, and water splashing hit me with the ambiance of a school playground during recess, not an army boot camp. Sliding back in my chaise, I realized that the hotshot teacher presented no threat to my irrepressible girl. I began to relax, unaware of the unwanted attention about to come *my* way at the end of the class.

While the other swimmers climbed out of the water, as instructed, my girls threw a party. Splashing, laughing, practicing holding their heads underwater, they were oblivious to teachers shouting, "Out of the pool!" The teachers might have assumed that the girls didn't understand, but I knew better.

Feeling chagrined, I rose from my chair shrieking, "Out! *Seychas!*" *Now*. Still no response. "Out *seychas*, or no *marozhina*!" That got their attention.

With the threat of no ice cream, their hearing improved. Lickety-split, they emerged from the pool. Vika draped a peach-colored towel over her head and shoulders and seated herself on my lap. Shivering, Maria snuggled beside me for warmth. Both girls eyed the vending machine standing outside the locker room doors.

Pinching the towel together under her chin, Vika looked up at me like a tiny saint draped in a terry cloth veil. "Gail, ice cream?" she asked in her sweetest voice. Maria sat up, waiting for my answer.

"Tomorrow will you come out of the pool when teachers say, 'Out'?" I asked.

They both promised, though I knew that promise was one that two nine-year-old swimming fish girls couldn't keep. Still, I filled their palms with quarters.

Each morning, Vika marched in like the Queen of Swimming 101. All smiles, she waved to her teacher and greeted him in English, undeterred by his cold shoulder. At the conclusion of the two-week class, she could swim in deep water *and* she still possessed her sweet innocence. I, too, was learning to swim. In the murky waters of parenthood.

CHAPTER 10

The Road to *Ozero* Chelan

W earing a determined smile and her hot pink Picasso-print spandex, Vika pulled a roller bag into the kitchen where I stood at the counter dicing garlic and shredding cheese, making a Russian egg salad for our trip to eastern Washington.

"*Ozero* Chelan six good morning!" she announced. Her breath carried the scents of chocolate, strategies, and exuberance. She wanted to be on the road to Lake Chelan at six in the morning.

"*Niet*. Too early." I still had a lot to do before I could put this long, busy day behind me, and I needed a good night's sleep. Rising at five to be on the road by six wouldn't work for me.

"Gail!" Vika stamped her bare foot on the floor. "*Po-zhal-uysta!*" she begged. *Pleeease*.

"You're excited."

"*Da*," she panted. Her frown disappeared.

"Is that *moy sumka*?" *My suitcase*? She grinned.

Vika knew that she could borrow almost anything of mine, that I'd give her the moon if I could. One day I had found her outdoors, dancing on the front deck, wearing one of my favorite skirts, a long, flowy number with beaded tassels and a bold print of bright colors that popped against a black background. The green, red, purple, yellow, and orange skirt swirled around her like a pandemonium of parrots. I would carry that vision of her—all color and joy—forever.

Now, as she stood in the kitchen, Vika set her jaw tight. Of the two girls, she was less volatile and more persevering, capable of badgering me until I caved. I felt relieved when Mike showed up with an empty cooler and plunked it down on the floor. He would take the pressure off me.

"Here you go." He lifted his cap and wiped sweat from his brow with the back of his hand. "Anything else?" He sounded weary.

What he really wanted, I knew, was for us to relax together before going to bed, instead of turning in completely exhausted. He didn't mind waiting until morning to finish preparations for a road trip. I, on the other hand, preferred to finish packing *before* bed. And, because I liked to come home to a clean, tidy house, I would have been delighted for Mike to vacuum the floors while I finished the salad and packing. Knowing we both were tired, I decided not to push it.

"Vika wants to leave at six in the morning," I said.

Mike's head spun in her direction. His flyaway eyebrows jumped, then froze in midair, yanking his eyes wide open. *Here comes the red light*, I thought, expecting him to say, *That ain't gonna happen.*

Vika saw it coming too, but not ready to concede, she turned her puppy-dog eyes on him and cocked her head. I could see Mike's mind searching for a way to say no without dampening her excitement.

"I'll tell you what," he said, smiling, "you can wake us when you wake up, as long as it isn't before six. But no alarm clock."

"No u-larm clock?" she asked, confused.

"No *bzzzzzzzzzzzzz*!" he explained, pointing to the clock on the microwave oven with his arm vibrating.

Surprise brightened her eyes. "Okay!" she agreed. Eager to share The Deal with Maria, Vika hurried off with the *sumka*.

"They won't wake up before eight," Mike predicted, sounding sure of himself. I wasn't so certain.

This most likely would be the girls' first visit to a lakeside resort. In Belarus, their family vacations involved pulling weeds and digging up potatoes at their *babushka's* house in Ukraine. To swim, they walked an hour to reach a small lake in the woods.

Lake Chelan, we had explained to the girls, was deep, icy cold, crystal clear, and over fifty miles long, like a giant dragon tail. The lakeside condominium we had rented had access to swimming pools, a water slide, rafts, paddleboats, and snow cones. Maria and Vika would have walked through fire to get there as soon as possible.

Now, as I mixed mayonnaise into the egg salad, a loud noise rose from the belly of the house. *Thunk! Thunk! Thunk! Thunk!*

"What's *that*?" Mike asked, his broad forehead collapsed into quizzical folds.

I knew without seeing. "It's Maria," I said. "She's dragging a roller bag up the stairs from the basement."

Still reeking of chlorine from her final swim class that morning, Maria appeared at the top of the stairs with an overnight bag, just as I had predicted. "Gail, I make," she said, hefting it onto her bed. She and Vika went to work packing swimsuits, stuffed animals, and favorite movies—*Pocahontas*, *Lion King*, and *101 Dalmatians*.

"Who wants *kukuruza*?" Mike hollered just as their bags were zipped closed.

Cheering, the girls and I streamed into the bedroom behind Mike. We all climbed onto the bed, with Mike and me leaning against pillows at the head of the bed, the girls facing us with their backs against the footboard. The giant bowl of salted popcorn sat in the center where everyone could reach in. With our feet and legs all tangled together, we savored that corn like every kernel was a tiny kiss.

"We're going to see snow in the Cascade Mountains," Mike told the girls.

"Snow? Now?" Vika couldn't imagine snow on the ground in the middle of summer.

"*Da*. The mountains are biiiiiig."

"How long *Ozero* Chelan?" Vika asked, wondering how long she'd have to sit in the car.

"*Chetyre den*, maybe more," I replied, thinking I had said four hours or more.

"*Chetyre den!*" Maria barked as though I had said we were going to walk across the mountains.

"No, no!" said Mike, realizing I'd misspoken. "*Chetyre* hours, *niet* days."

"Gail!" said Maria in a deep scolding voice. She and Vika then lit into me for telling them it would take four days or more to reach Chelan. On and on they chastised me, as though I had committed a despicable crime. Finally, I broke in.

"*Izvinite menya!*" *Excuse me*. I apologized in an exaggerated, offended tone. "*Ya niet gavorit Russkiy!*" *I don't speak Russian*. Though the twins understood what I meant, I had mangled those words too. They collapsed on the bed in fits of snorts and laughter, scattering popcorn everywhere.

When the last *kukuruza* kernel disappeared, we brushed salt off the sheets, and the twins brushed and flossed their teeth, then crawled into bed, though they were too excited to sleep. They began to sing at the top of their lungs.

"Go to sleep!" Mike hollered. They giggled and squealed. "Now!" The singing continued.

"Girls! Go to sleep!" I tried to sound fierce. More singing and giggles. "You're going to wake the neighbors."

It was a long while before they tuckered themselves out and silence filled the house. Six hours later, at 5:00 a.m., I heard them dash from their bedroom to the kitchen.

"Mike," I whispered, "they're checking the clock." His eyes opened slowly, as though he might still be dreaming. The pitter-patter headed from the kitchen to our room.

"Shhhh," he answered. His eyelids floated closed. We both knew that if either of us stirred, the girls would jump on the bed to get the show on the road. With eyes closed, I tried not to move or twitch. Our strategy worked. Whispering, the twins went back to bed. But not for long.

Fifteen minutes later they checked the time again. While we tried to doze, they carried on this way until five minutes before six. Then, unable to restrain themselves another five minutes, they scuttled into our room and climbed onto the foot of our bed singing, "Good mor-ning!"

An hour later we were on the road and the girls fell asleep in the car. Mike and I were enjoying the quiet drive until, climbing the foothills into the Cascade Mountains, the car began to wobble. I looked at Mike as my shoulders tightened.

"What's going on?"

"Flat tire." Gripping the wheel, Mike braked slowly and steered toward the shoulder of the old two-lane highway.

"Do we have a spare?"

"Nope." The Camry ground to a halt, awakening the girls with a start.

"We're okay," I reassured them, unclasping my seat belt. "We have a flat tire. Get out on this side. Stay away from the road!"

Mumbling expletives under his breath, Mike pulled all our gear from the trunk to find the jack. Maria appeared to be even more troubled than Mike.

"American *mashina*! American *mashina*!" Maria spewed. Wearing white platform gym shoes with soles as thick as bricks, she ranted and raved on the side of the road, kicking up dirt and gravel. I had purchased those shoes at her insistence and against my own better judgment, afraid she would twist her ankle or fall and injure herself. Now, I held my breath until she calmed down.

Through Maria's eyes, our pile of belongings tossed on the ground must have looked like a heap of broken dreams. In her idealized version of America, this catastrophe couldn't happen. She must have thought our trip would end then and there, on Highway 2. She couldn't know that, with AAA road service, we'd have a new tire delivered and be back on the road to Chelan again in a couple of hours. That wasn't how life worked in Belarus.

Though the spectacle made me want to laugh, I knew better than to reveal my amusement during Maria's moment of disillusion, or to remind her that it was a Japanese car, not American. Mike, now fighting lug nuts, was in no mood for humor either. So I gathered up my books, a notebook, and a blanket, and went scouting for a quiet spot in the shade. Vika trailed me to a grassy area. There we spread the blanket, creating a little secret sanctuary on the edge of the wilderness. Maria joined us when her short-lived squall blew over.

While I tried to catch up on journal writing, birds called from the trees, and the twins entertained themselves by walking around with books balanced on their heads. They took slow, careful steps, their backs straight and chins forward like prim and proper mannequins.

Engrossed in simple pleasure, surrounded by trees and ferns, I forgot we were next to a highway with logging trucks groaning uphill. Somewhere in the distance water trickled. Transported to an old world the girls knew well, I delighted in their ability to entertain themselves—with Barbara Kingsolver and Kathleen Norris books perched on their heads, and no battery-operated devices. When they tired of that game, they wandered off while I wrote.

"Don't go far, girls!"

"Okay, Gail."

Not a minute later, they were screaming, "Gail! Mike! Look! Look!"

Panic shot through me like a meteor. Were those screams of joy or terror? I couldn't be sure. Visions of bears and dead bodies flooded my mind as I flew to my feet.

"I'm coming!" I yelled. My pulse throbbed in my head as I ran toward their voices. Behind a pile of brush, I found them standing by a tower of old tires. Thinking we could replace our flat tire with one they'd found, they were beaming with pride and astonishment.

Unable to stop myself, I burst out laughing. "Tires no good," I said. "Broken." Their faces sagged with disappointment.

By the time AAA rescued us with a new tire and we reloaded the trunk, all of us were tired and fidgety.

"How long *Ozero* Chelan?" Vika asked. Maria asked again five minutes later.

With the Columbia River on one side of us and a wall of jagged rock on the other, we followed Highway 2 for miles. After a few more bends in the road, we saw in the distance vast sun-burned hillsides dotted with green irrigated vineyards and orchards. A glimmering blue ribbon, *Ozero* Chelan unraveled across the valley into a dream of mountains and sky.

"Maria, look!" Vika cried.

"Ohmigod!" said Maria, using a phrase I often used. Hearing it tumble from her mouth, I cringed.

With white wispy clouds drifting across a brilliant blue sky and the sun bouncing off the lake, it looked like we were approaching heaven. Taking it all in, the girls could hardly speak. Their auras had turned ecstatic pink.

CHAPTER 11

Dr. No and The Boss

Undaunted by glacier water, my beautiful swimming fish girls plunged into Lake Chelan with the ease of walking into a steamy *banya*.

"*Gorka!*" Maria hollered, pointing at the slide attached to a raft anchored in deep water.

From the moment she and Vika had spotted the slide from the balcony of our condo, they could think about nothing else. They shimmied into swimsuits as fast as they could and urged us to hurry. Fresh out of swimming classes, they were possessed with the chutzpah of Olympic swimmers. Now, I worried Maria would head to deep water without a life jacket and without waiting for Mike and me.

"*Niet!* You wait!" I yelled back. Mike and I had agreed that we would all swim to the raft together and the girls would have to wear life jackets. They had learned to swim in a warm pool, not a choppy, frigid lake two thousand feet deep in some places. We weren't taking any chances.

"Gail, *gorka*!" Vika whined. The distress in her voice told me her patience was growing thin.

Gulping a deep breath, I launched myself into the crystal-clear water. It set off a pins-and-needles sensation in me from limb to limb. Recovering from the shock, I called to Mike.

"Come on! They can't wait much longer." Two life vests dangled on my arm.

Standing at the edge of the water with hands crossed over his slightly hairy chest, shoulders hunched, he turned toward me with questioning eyes. *Do I have to?*

"You'd better jump in before the girls get to you," I warned. They were already headed toward him, hooting, hollering, and scooping water with their cupped hands.

"Mike! *Plavat! Gorka!*" *Swim. Slide.*

"*Niet!* No splashing!" Mike yelled. His begging multiplied their delight. Screaming and laughing, they blasted him with numbing liquid pellets until he dove in.

"Okay, Gail, *davay!*" cried Maria. *Come on!*

"First you need to put on life vests," I said, handing one to each girl. Vika, still a bit uncertain of her own endurance, slipped one on and snapped it closed. She would have worn snow pants and hiking boots, if necessary, to swim to that raft. But Maria refused.

"I *no* vest!"

"*Da*, Maria. You can take it off on the raft," I promised.

"Me no."

Mike and I exchanged glances. I could read his mind. We both were thinking, *Here we go again.* "Me No" had become Maria's favorite refrain, so much so that, privately, we sometimes referred to her as Doctor No.

"You have to wear your life vest, Maria." Mike's voice sounded stern.

"*Niet!*" She folded her arms over her chest. Her lower lip curled.

"Come on, Maria. We can't go until you put it on." I tried to sound calm, though my patience was now wearing thin.

Ready for a standoff, Maria bent one knee, shifted her

weight, and tightened her arms. Trying to reason with her wasn't working. Feeling helpless, I fantasized about putting her on the next plane to Moscow. But, in my heart, I wanted the four of us on the raft together. I was about to threaten to call Victor or write to Zoya, threats which I had used successfully in the past, when Vika stepped into the fray, as she often did when she suspected Maria's behavior would cause her to suffer too. Her conniptions had been so successful in influencing Maria to change her behavior that they had earned Vika a private nickname too—The Boss.

With daggers in her eyes, The Boss flew into a tirade I couldn't understand. The dark, threatening tone suggested Dr. No would wear the vest or face nasty consequences she would regret for the remainder of her life. As an afterthought, Vika threw in additional consequences, in English.

"No life vest, no *marozhina and* no computer, *da* Gail?"

"*Da*," I agreed, trying not to laugh. Mike and I had often held the threat of no ice cream over Maria's head, but this was a first for withholding computer privileges. The Boss's strategy worked.

Sour-faced, Maria snatched the vest from me and buckled herself in. Then, like magic, her mood shifted from sullen to scintillating, as though her defiance had been carried away on the wind. Buoyed by the sudden shift, our pod set off as though the dust-up had never happened. After standing in the blazing sun, the water now felt cool and refreshing, a maiden voyage I would cherish.

The moment we landed on the raft, the girls ditched the vests, scrambled up the ladder, and careened down the *gorka*. Screaming, they disappeared, one after the other, into the water's dark depths as though Chelan had swallowed them whole. After their heads popped out of the water I realized I'd been holding my breath. Mike and I dangled our feet in the water and cheered for the girls until their lips turned blue.

In a purple glow spreading across the water as the sun reached for the horizon, we headed leisurely back to shore. As we glided in, the shallow water now seemed almost tepid. Time slowed. A transcendent oneness with Mike, the girls, the sky, and the water poured into me. Vika clung to me like a happy barnacle, kissing my face, then pushing away with our fingers clasped. When our arms reached full extension, she pulled me back to her, smooched, then pushed away again. Ebbing and flowing, we were gentle waves of a poem. Maria spun around us like a satellite in orbit, coming close for an occasional kiss, then pushing off again to exercise her independence. The dark days of fertility treatment, pregnancy loss, and depression seemed worlds away. I slipped into a snow-globe universe where, instead of whirling crystals of ice, a swirl of love surrounded Mike, the twins, and me.

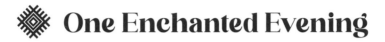 One Enchanted Evening

A hush settled over the lake as the sun dropped behind the mountains. The Wapato Point beehive of condominiums became quiet as dozens of families settled in for the night. Maria and Vika climbed into pajamas after a shower, planning to fall asleep watching *The Lion King* for the umpteenth time. I, too, had settled in to savor the end of the day when Mike burst into the room with a proposal.

"Let's walk under the stars!" His excitement created a second wind.

The girls' ears perked up. Their eyes darted from Mike to me.

"*Poshli!*" I said. *Let's go.* "Put your sweatshirts on over your pajamas, girls."

Like a gaze of raccoons on the prowl, we headed down a dark trail. Possessed with an eye for beautiful landscapes and nature's tiny details, Vika took the lead. Earlier that day she had stopped to admire a marching band of a mama and baby quails, all festooned with head plumes. Now, wielding flashlights, she and Maria, their hair still dripping wet from the shower, led us toward the water.

With no warning, Vika halted. "*Chto eto?*" she asked. *What is this?* We all squeezed in around her. On the dirt

path, shining under the beam of her light, we saw a narrow
trail of goop.

Mike bent down for a closer view. "Ooze from a slug,"
he said.

Vika was puzzled. "What slug?"

"Fat, slimy critters that come out at night to eat," Mike
said in a spooky voice. "Some are small, like this . . ." He
spread his thumb and index finger three inches apart. "And
some are giant yellow slugs, like *this*!" His hands sprang a
foot apart, startling the girls. His wicked laugh made their
eyes grow wide. Worry lines formed on Maria's face.

"Mike! Stop scaring them," I huffed. "Mike cuckoo," I
reassured the girls, using our word for describing anything
we considered outlandish or goofy.

The girls smirked at Mike as if to say, *You can't fool us!
We knew all along you were kidding.*

"Slugs won't hurt you," I continued. "They eat plants.
Poshli." I hoped my nonchalance concealed my own repul-
sion for the Pacific Northwest's ubiquitous gastropod
mollusk. Like worms on steroids, with buggy eyes perched
on the tips of tentacles and a suction cup for a foot, they
gave me the heebie-jeebies. I'd heard that human skin burned
on contact with the sticky mucus that coats their bodies.
Whether that was a fact or an old wives' tale, I wasn't sure,
but I didn't want to take any chances.

"If you see a slug, don't touch it!" I warned the girls.
"We don't want to hurt them," I added, not wanting to
alarm the twins again.

As we continued on the path, Maria now took the lead,
moving in slow motion with her eyes glued to the ground.
I quickened my step to catch up with her so that I could
surreptitiously keep watch too. Playing in my mind was
a ridiculous scene of the girls or me slipping on a giant
slug the size of a sausage, falling to the ground, screaming

bloody murder, legs melting and burning. The hideous image stopped when Maria reached the sandy beach and something caught her eye.

"Gail, look." She'd found a child's book and hair ribbon in the sand beside the picnic table. "Maybe little girl cry. Maybe mama mad," Maria said with concern.

"Let's put them here on the table, in case she comes back for them tomorrow," I suggested.

Squatting beside the water with her knees pressed to her chest, Vika called to us. "Look! Look!" Her tone sounded urgent.

Mike, Maria, and I scuttled over and peered into the lake where a shaft of light from Vika's flashlight shot through the water. Rocks and pebbles burst to life in shades of green, blue, gray, and purple. Algae clung to stones like dozens of layers of peeling paint. Beyond the lighted galaxy, inky darkness lurked.

Maria squatted next to her sister. "*Krasivaya*," she cooed. *Beautiful.*

Overhead, stars dusted the sky. The night air carried the occasional sound of a faraway laugh, a door closing, a plate dropped on a counter. Across the water stood a silent silhouette of mountains like granite curtains.

Maria sliced the water with a second ray of light. As the crystal-clear aquatic universe expanded, intriguing patterns and fusions of matter appeared on shiny rocks like secret codes written millions of years ago. Those rocks told the story of volcanoes erupting, mountains rising, glaciers melting—cataclysmic events that had given birth to Lake Chelan. Awed by that story of creation, I realized it echoed our story too. The eruption of a disastrous explosion led to the rise of a dormant dream and had brought us together. Now Lake Chelan was a part of our story. I wanted our story written in those stones too, as lasting evidence of our moment there.

After gazing into the nocturnal underwater world, we perched on a picnic table like four gulls enjoying a hint of breeze. Mike snuggled up beside me on the tabletop and put his arm around my shoulders. With their backs to us, the girls sat on the bench between our feet. As we gazed out over the lake in silence, I recalled the language and cultural differences that had stood between us as we took our first steps together on this journey. It had been messy and awkward. But we had kept our hearts open and taken risks that had blended our differences together like a pot of tasty soup. Now, two summers and a dozen letters into our journey, I wanted to sit there under the stars together until I grew old. At the same time, I felt the sadness of an approaching ending.

Soon we would return to Seattle for the girls' last two weeks in the United States. I knew from the previous summer that they would long for their mama, papa, and sister as the end drew near. Every day would be chaotic and busy, shopping for vitamins, winter coats, and presents for the family. There would be final visits with friends and neighbors. As I grieved the inevitable changes on the way, Vika broke the silence.

"No more America?" Sadness hung in the air along with her question. Would we invite them back the next summer?

Caught off guard, neither Mike nor I knew how to reply. There was no easy answer, and so many complications Vika couldn't understand. I took a breath. I knew Mike must be feeling the same squeezing in his heart that I felt. Searching for a response, I combed my fingers through Vika's hair.

Recently, we had learned that the program was a target of harassment by the Belarusian government and could be forced to disband. That wasn't an issue we discussed with the girls. I didn't know if their parents were even aware of these threats.

There were obstacles on our side too. My mother's health was deteriorating. Unable to continue caring for my father at home, she had recently moved him to an Alzheimer's care facility. Mike's brother was fighting mesothelioma, a cancer caused by exposure to asbestos. Though they all lived across the country, in Michigan, Mike and I were involved in their care and support. The unpredictability of their needs made planning difficult. Our physical, emotional, and financial resources were stretched. The last thing I wanted was to make a promise to the girls without knowing for certain whether we could follow through.

"We hope we can invite you back next summer, but we'll have to wait and see," I replied. It was the kind of response I hated—a cop-out. I felt grateful Vika's back was turned toward me so we didn't have to make eye contact.

"Me like Gail. Me like Mike. Me like Gail's home." Her appeal was soft and morose. As her expression of love and attachment registered in my bones, a bittersweet wave of affection rolled through me. I kept stroking her thick, sun-bleached hair while my heart pulled apart.

"We like to have you in our home," I said. "I'm going to miss you girls." At the same time, I wondered if the twins' visits might have unintended consequences. What seeds were we planting? Would temporary immersions in a materialistic culture set them up to believe that we could change their standard of living in Belarus? Would they one day resent us for our wealth? Still, the only direction I knew to follow was the one that said we belong to each other.

As Vika and I spoke of our future, Maria quietly dragged her feet back and forth in the sand. I didn't know how to read her silence. Were goodbyes difficult for her? Or did she resent having to leave her home and family for the summer? Could that explain her cantankerous moments when I wanted to put Dr. No on the first flight back to Moscow?

Still hoping for some assurance that we would see each other again, Vika asked, "Maybe Mike, Gail come to Zalessie?"

Her heartfelt invitation brought tears to my eyes. And I felt sad because I knew, the instant she spoke the name of their village, she had been transported to a different world.

Though Mike and I both dreamed of one day meeting the girls' family and experiencing their culture, there were numerous impediments we had to consider. My health issues made me hesitant to travel to places where I couldn't avoid potentially disabling environmental toxins. What if there was a leaky gas stove in Zoya and Ivan's apartment? What if the linens were laundered with scented products? How would I avoid foods containing gluten and dairy? What if family members wore perfume or aftershave? The language barrier would make explaining my needs difficult if not impossible and increase the risk of offending our hosts, something I wished to avoid at all costs. In Belarus, my options would be limited. These were risks I wasn't yet ready to take. Nor was I ready to face the Cold War fears that still lingered deep within me.

As Vika's question hung in the air, I felt strangled by its complications. Unable to speak, I signaled Mike with a pleading glance to address this question.

"Maybe someday," he said, though he didn't sound hopeful. "But it would be hard for Gail with her illness." The girls understood my need to avoid exposures to fragrances and chemicals and seemed to accept that as a sufficient answer.

Though I didn't want to talk about their leaving, I wanted to make room for their unspoken longings. "You're thinking about going home," I said, opening that door.

"*Da*. We go Babushka. Mama and Papa drive *mashina*," Vika answered wistfully. I imagined the family packed in their little car as they made the twelve-hour drive to Babushka's village in Ukraine.

"Papa like Babushka *sobaka*, Jack," said Maria, joining the conversation. I'd seen pictures of Babushka's dog, Jack Daniels.

"Papa kiss Jack like baby," Vika laughed. "Mama no like Jack *rarararrrr*!" Her imitation of the dog barking made it clear that Jack Daniels was a tough little bugger.

"Babushka sing, Papa . . ." Maria's narrow body swayed back and forth, her fingers dancing as she opened and closed her bent arms.

"Babushka sings and Papa plays an accordion?" I remembered seeing an accordion sitting on the ground in the picture taken of the family in front of Babushka's little white house with the blue trim and door.

"*Da.*"

"Mama *yi* Papa dance," Vika continued.

I pictured Ivan sweeping Zoya across a dimly lit room perfumed with dill and garlic, the girls dancing solo, and Babushka, with a flowered headscarf tied under her chin, singing a Ukrainian folk song. I, too, wanted to dance in that room.

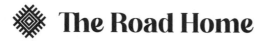 The Road Home

It was a sizzling ninety degrees when we said goodbye to *Ozero* Chelan and headed home on the northern route. The mountainous North Cascades Highway climbed steadily between granite walls and rugged peaks. As our elevation rose, the temperature dropped dramatically. In the distance, snow clung to rocky ledges and waterfalls dangled from cliffs like frozen white shoelaces.

At 5,476 feet above sea level, we stopped to stretch our legs, enjoy the view, and use the facilities at Washington Pass Overlook Park. A white blanket covered the ground.

"Snow?" Vika asked, incredulously.

"*Da!*"

A frosty wind slapped our faces when we emerged from the car. Still dressed for the ninety-degree temperature we'd left in Chelan, the girls and I hustled to the restroom. When we came back out, a snowball suddenly hurtled by us, barely missing Vika's arm. Startled, we stopped in our tracks to survey the grounds, in search of the culprit who had targeted us.

"Mike!" cried Maria. He was standing under a towering tree with a devilish grin on his face and a second snowball ready to fly.

The girls took the bait. Wearing shorts and flip-flops, they scooped snow with their bare hands, laughing and screaming. An August snowball fight ensued, strange and madcap as a Mardi Gras parade in Siberia.

I skirted around the line of fire, headed to the car, and pulled sweatshirts out of our luggage. "Come get your coats," I called. No response. Snowballs were flying in every direction. "Mike! The girls are going to freeze!" I said, raising my voice. "Put on your sweatshirts and let's go out to the viewpoint."

With chattering teeth and a quivering jaw, Vika finally ran to the car. Red splotches covered her legs where they'd been smacked with snow. She pulled her sweatshirt over her head and shivered. When Maria arrived, holding herself in a bear hug, I handed her a sweatshirt.

"I no," she said.

"We're going out to the viewpoint, Maria. You need something warm."

"I *mashina*."

"No, you can't sit in the car alone, Maria. Come on."

"I no walk," she said, opening the car door.

"It's not far. And it's beautiful! You'll see," I said, trying to coax Dr. No. She slid into the back seat and closed the door. I rolled my eyes, and Mike's hand floated to my lower back to steer me toward the trailhead.

"You and Vika go out to the viewpoint. I'll stay here close to the parking lot, where I can see the car."

Holding hands, Vika and I stepped into a primeval world. Gray mountain jays swung from tree to tree squawking noisily as we meandered along the path. The intoxicating scent of cedar perfumed the air.

Near the edge of a cliff, behind a guardrail, we sat huddled together for warmth on a flat-topped granite boulder. Like baby eagles nesting in a treetop, eye-to-eye with Liberty Bell's snowy peaks, we gaped at miles of vastness. *This is my temple*, I thought, sitting on a hard stone pew. Waves of blue and violet mountains flowed to infinity.

"Ohhhh, *krasivaya*," Vika murmured. *Beautiful.* The gentle rise and fall of her breath aligned with mine.

At this nexus of heaven and earth, I experienced time and boundaries fading until Vika and I were no longer visitors or spectators, we were part of a deep and beautiful mystery. Then Vika began to shiver, and I realized we needed to leave. She was cold, and Mike had said he wanted to be out of the mountains before nightfall.

"Time to go," I said. Taking a last look at the holy place, I hoped Vika would stow this memory away and one day share it with her children and grandchildren. As we headed back, I imagined her telling her little ones the story of the mountains. *It was like a dream. We were high in the clouds, sitting on a rock surrounded by ancient trees over two hundred feet tall.* I pictured her children's eyes shining with possibility as she told them stories and sang them to sleep with "Colors of the Wind," a song about the lives and spirits of rocks and trees and wild creatures that she and Maria learned from watching *Pocahontas*, one of their favorite Disney films, over and over that summer.

When we reached the parking area, Maria emerged from the car wearing her sweatshirt. "I go!" she said cheerily.

Part of me wanted to tell her she had missed that boat. At the same time, I wanted the little rebel I loved to have the same experience of awe Vika and I had shared. Though beautiful forests are abundant in Belarus—including a part of the oldest and largest primeval forest in Europe—the country was mostly flat. I was afraid Maria might never have another opportunity to sit on the edge of a mountain, more than a mile above sea level, face-to-face with infinity, mystery, and moss. The view from inside the car didn't do it justice.

"Okay," I said. "Let's go!"

Mike's eyes darted to me and his brows furrowed. I knew he wanted to make it down the mountain before dark, and he didn't think I should reinforce Maria's earlier defiance by making a second trip to the viewpoint.

"This is a rare opportunity to attune her DNA to nature's frequency," I explained. "And I want Maria to know and tell the story of a place so pristine and close to heaven."

Mike capitulated to my lofty goals, though I'm sure his expectations were far more realistic than mine. On this outing, there would be no alchemical impact on Maria's DNA. No spiritual awakening.

When the four of us reached the viewpoint, daredevil Maria pressed her back against the fence along the cliff, threw her arms up, and tipped her head back, pretending to fall over the edge of the earth.

"Take picture, Gail!" she hollered, enjoying the thrill. Though the fence was secure, my heart raced, and I wanted to drag her back to the car.

"No. We have to get going. *Now!* Before it's dark!" I snapped.

"So much for her DNA," Mike said wryly.

"I need to leave before my heart stops," I hissed. Apparently, the whole troop realized I meant business. Without another word, they followed me back down the path.

Golden rays spiked the sky when we headed out on the highway. Halfway down the mountain, we encountered a roadblock and followed a detour through a forest carpeted with sword ferns, Oregon grape, rhododendrons, and sorrel. The narrow road carried us deep into a Tolkien world under a canopy of old-growth fir and hemlock. Though we never stopped, it seemed as though we were at a standstill in a fairy tale. The twins began to sing folk songs. Their harmonies carried through the woods like sirens calling. Listening to their soulful voices, I wanted to lie on a blanket under a tree and fall asleep to dream the potent dreams of wild places.

Twilight descended when we rejoined the highway. Faint swirls of light tinted the clouds with Easter egg colors. Vika's and Maria's voices faded out as though an invisible conductor had ever so slowly lowered her baton.

"Maybe Mama *pismo*," said Vika, sounding a bit sad and sleepy. She was hoping a letter from her mother would be waiting in Seattle when we got home.

I too hoped there would be one, because I didn't want the girls to feel disappointed, homesick, or hurt. "Maybe today Mama reading letters from you," I said. We had mailed their letters to Zoya before leaving for Chelan. It took a week or longer for letters to reach Zalessie. Some never arrived.

"In Zalessie, we light candle when *pismo* come from America," said Vika.

"Mama, Papa, Elina, Vika, I sit in circle. Mama say *pismo* so I and Vika no fight," Maria laughed.

"Mama reads the letters out loud so you girls don't fight over who reads them first?" I pictured the family circle, in a room lit by candlelight, as Zoya read our letters, typed in Cyrillic by a translator in Seattle.

"*Da.*"

"Mama say Mike, Gail *dome* in Zalessie," Vika added. I understood that, when our letters were read, they felt our presence in their house in Zalessie.

"Sometimes rain, candles," said Maria. "I scared."

"You light candles when there's a storm and the lights go out? And it's scary?"

"*Da.*"

"Maria many scared in Zalessie. Maybe no rain, stomach hurt," said Vika.

Now I realized that the night fears troubling Maria in Seattle had their roots in Zalessie. What dark thoughts worried her? What spoken and unspoken dangers did she sense? I remembered my own childhood of nightmares and stomach distress arising from my mother sleeping with a gun under her pillow when Dad was away, and the nightly television news: *Russian missiles in Cuba ready to strike. Race riots. Ku Klux Klan.*

Would the legacy of fear never end?

A brief but peaceful quiet settled over us. Soon my thoughts began to drift back to the girls' imminent departure. I felt twinges of grief and fear of the void their absence would leave. Then out of the blue, Vika remarked, "Change is good." It was a line I knew she had borrowed from *The Lion King*. Her casual proclamation struck me as so hilarious and ironic that I burst out laughing.

"*Chto*, Gail?" she asked, surprised by my reaction. "*Chto*, change is good?" *What does it mean?*

"To start something new is good," I tried to explain. "Not repeating the same old thing."

Memory by memory, song by song, we were building a legacy of stories. Stories of journeying, expansiveness, change, and a global family making their way home.

Part Four:

1999

CHAPTER 14

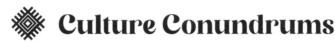 **Culture Conundrums**

"Open it! It's for you!" said Michelle, Mike's now fourteen-year-old niece from Arizona. Four years older than the twins, she was like a big sister they had adored ever since their first visit. Her blonde silky hair hung above her shoulders in tight waves, and her rosy cheeks glowed with excitement as she waited for the girls to open the suitcase filled with clothes and accessories she'd outgrown.

Michelle had traveled alone to Seattle to welcome Vika and Maria at the airport with us when they arrived for their third summer visit. Despite her eagerness, the twins weren't about to open Michelle's suitcase until they had completed their own gift-giving mission.

"Wait, please," said Maria.

Vika unzipped the familiar black duffel and the bag breathed open with a sigh. The ritual began with candy for Michelle to share with her brothers at home and a dish to take back to her mother.

Next, the twins presented me with a hand-embroidered *rushnyk*, a traditional Ukrainian ritual cloth, similar to a long table runner, used for blessings, protection, and honoring sacred events from birth to death.

"Babushka make," said Vika with reverence. In Ukrainian culture, a house with no *rushnyk* is not a home.

Holding the treasure, I could feel Babushka's spirit of generosity and love embedded in the traditional motifs she had stitched on both ends with bold black, red, green, and yellow threads. I pictured her sewing on cold winter nights in the little blue-trimmed house I'd seen in a photograph. And I sensed the satisfaction she must have felt when she finished the piece and entrusted her granddaughters to carry it with them to America.

"Krasivaya!" Beautiful.

Zoya had also sent a gift that I would cherish—a porcelain figurine of a woman kneeling in front of a child, her arms open, waiting to embrace the little one reaching for her, their blue eyes locked in a loving gaze. Through the cool pearlescent finish of that powerful maternal symbol, I felt seen, known, and connected to Zoya, a woman I'd never met, separated from me by an ocean and two continents. Still coming to terms with three pregnancy losses, I felt my understanding of fertility shifting as I held her gift in my hands. My heart was singing.

After the girls emptied the black duffel, Michelle invited them to open the suitcase filled with surprises for them. "Now," she said, with a sweeping gesture of her hand, "it's your turn."

Feeling awkward on the receiving end, the twins shyly sat on the floor beside Michelle, opened the hinges, and lifted the lid. Out popped a stuffed lion with fuzzy gold hair.

"Simba!" cried Vika, swooping the animal into her arms. She and Maria both adored the star of *The Lion King*.

Vika quickly claimed the prize, with no protest from Maria. When it came to ownership, the girls always partnered. That endearing trait always astonished me. Though Vika often played the heavy-handed older sibling—born just thirty minutes before Maria—they didn't seem to view themselves as two individuals with separate boundaries and possessions. Accustomed to sharing the same womb, same breast, same clothes, same toys, and same bed, separateness might have struck them as completely unnatural, if not impossible. Perhaps the history and practice of collectivism in Belarus also played a part.

After the Simba moment, Maria pulled a collection of arm bangles out of the suitcase and slipped them over her wrist. Vika put together an ensemble with a few items that caught her eye, and tried it on. With her shoulders pulled back and her face shining like a pearl, she strutted around the room modeling flowered tights, a gray T-shirt with USA in big red letters splashed across her chest, a faux leopard-skin handbag swinging from her arm, and white heeled sandals that *click, click, clicked* across the hardwood floor.

Oozing with satisfaction, the girls showed no interest in perusing all that still remained in the gift bag. The bounty was more than two young girls could process, and more than they could ever use or want, though I didn't understand that at the time.

Every summer in Seattle, Vika and Maria acquired a mountain of possessions—new clothes, shoes, and other items we bought in stores, gently used goods we found at yard sales, and contributions from friends, family, and neighbors who were eager to share their abundance with the girls. We failed to take into account the practical realities of living in small spaces, as most Europeans do, where storage is limited, and laundry is often hand-washed and hung to dry. We didn't yet realize that not everyone wants or needs more than a few changes of clothing.

I'd practiced recycling since before it was adopted as a necessary effort to save the planet. My mother and sister had introduced me to hunting for yard sale treasures that didn't break the bank, a form of entertainment that supported my environmental values. It never occurred to me that this was another form of overconsumption, or that I might corrupt the twins by encouraging them to seek pleasure from shopping.

Mike and I assumed that anything we sent to Zalessie that the twins' family couldn't use would be given away or sold for extra income. Years later, while visiting the girls in Eastern Europe, we would inadvertently learn that wasn't how it worked there.

That future day, the twins would take us to pick strawberries outside their late maternal grandmother's house in a tiny Ukrainian village. Except on occasions when their aunt from Kyiv visited the village, the two-room house sat empty. After our bowl was filled with berries, the girls took us inside. The room we entered was stuffy and dark. A narrow shaft of light slipped in through a curtained window. In the shadows stood a single piece of furniture, a hefty dark wood armoire, its doors flung open, the shelves piled high with clothing. A stray shirt sleeve dangled as if trying to escape. Mounds of clothes and toys sat on the floor in the eerie warehouse. *What is this?* I wondered.

"America," Vika explained with a single word.

Stunned, I stared at all we had sent to Belarus over the years. Mike and I exchanged glances of surprise and confusion. A feeling of shame rose from my belly. I felt like a foolish American. The goods we and others had bestowed upon the girls with love and concern now reeked of overconsumption. I couldn't imagine why the girls' family hadn't given away or sold things the kids had outgrown. Had they felt obligated to keep every gift they received? Why was it all stored in Ukraine, not Belarus?

In that room, staring at the face of materialism, I felt unable to voice my questions and discomfort. Talking about money was taboo, particularly with the economic disparity between us. Standing in that awkward situation, I felt that any conversation I began would lead to forbidden territory. And, because I still hadn't learned to converse in Russian, I worried the language barrier would make any attempt to talk about it even more difficult and confusing. I reckoned it was not worth the potential harm to our relationship, so I remained silent.

By not voicing my feelings, I missed the opportunity for intimacy and understanding that surfaced much later when I asked Maria about the mysterious room in her grandmother's house. That simple inquiry relieved me of years of unnecessary self-recrimination.

Maria explained that the storehouse of goods served the entire extended family as a lending bank. It was headquartered in Ukraine, she said, because their cousins all lived there.

"We need to help everyone. My sisters and cousins, sometimes friends, go to this house, take what they need. Now *we* have children. We take for our children." Anything still in good condition after it was used went back on the shelf to be borrowed by someone else.

Her understanding of interdependence reminded me of the Seventh Generation Principle embraced by indigenous people: Every decision made must consider how it will impact descendants seven generations into the future.

When I realized the recycling of our gifts continued after more than ten years, I saw those stacks of clothes and toys from a different perspective. Each of those gifts represented acts of love that had set in motion ripples of generosity and care on a different continent.

When Vika strutted around the room clicking her heels that day on her third trip to America, I never envisioned that there would come a time when the girls' children or their cousins' children might carry that same purse or wear the clothes she flaunted. What I saw was a girl with an artistic eye who knew what she wanted.

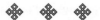

Later that summer of 1999, Vika accompanied me to a shop where I went to purchase a greeting card. There, she found and fell in love with an exquisite journal. "Gail, look!" she said, petting the hand-carved leather binding.

"Beautiful," I agreed. "Is very expensive. Sixty dollars. Put it back, please."

Though Vika's desires were not excessive, they could be persistent. I wanted to explain to her that this was not a book for children, and I'd be happy to purchase a notebook suited to her needs. But the language barrier between us made that kind of conversation impossible. And the store didn't carry notebooks suitable for ten-year-olds.

"I like," she said with a hint of pleading. She was burning with desire.

"I know. I'm sorry. Put it back," I said, loath to disappoint her.

Clutching the book, she didn't move. A knot twisted around my spine when I saw her grief-stricken eyes.

"We need to go."

Vika's face dropped like a stone in water. Reluctantly, she returned the journal to the display table and followed me to the register where I paid for a card. Her disappointment still weighed on me when we left the store.

A few days later I purchased back-to-school shoes for the girls. Paying at the register, I could see the wheels spinning in Vika's brain.

"Two shoes, sixty dollars. One book, sixty dollars," she remarked as we walked out the door.

"*Da*," I replied, slipping my arm over her shoulder. I thought we had turned a corner in the world of finances. But consumerism would continue to taunt us that summer.

Mike suggested we give the girls an allowance. That was

how our parents had taught us the value of money and how to make choices. We agreed to give the girls a weekly allowance of five dollars each as long as they made their bed each morning and helped with a few chores—both of which they already did without being asked.

With their allowance in their pockets, the girls and I roamed the neighborhood in search of yard sales on Saturday mornings. I kept an eye out for roller skates and other recreational equipment for them; it made no sense to pay for new equipment they would use for only one summer. Vika liked to buy stuffed animals and purses in mint condition, priced at 25 or 50 cents. Maria was partial to stuffed animals, jewelry, and trinkets to take home to friends and family. Pawing through an assortment of ladies' accessories at one house, Vika discovered something she considered a special treasure: a mink scarf. Holding the old fur wrap up by its tail, she beamed as though she'd just won the lottery.

Repulsed by the mink's head and claws dangling toward the ground, my first thought was, *That dead, beady-eyed animal isn't going home in my car!*

"Very interesting," I replied, after a pause. My tone lacked even a smidgen of enthusiasm.

"I buy!"

Now, I was flummoxed. Should I educate Vika about animal rights issues and veto her purchase? Or was that over-the-top ridiculous?

I decided I was taking social responsibility too far. It wasn't as if she was going on safari or poaching elephant tusks. That mink had been dead fifty years or more before Vika's birth. Buying it would keep it out of a landfill for at least a while longer. I gave her the green light.

Later that afternoon, while walking through the house, I caught a glimpse of Vika outside on the deck, blowing bubbles. She was wearing shorts, a T-shirt, and baggy socks, with the creepy mink wrapped around her neck. I wanted to freeze that comical, adorable moment for a thousand years.

"You are a ragtag queen!" I pronounced. "I want a picture painted of you to hang on my wall!" Her face broke into a smile.

One Saturday, Maria stormed into the house, sweaty hair plastered to her head, the five-dollar bill Mike had given her earlier that morning now crumpled in her hand. The air around her bristled and her jaw was set. She slapped the money down on the dining room table so hard that the crystal goblets tinkled in the china cabinet.

"This you!" she yelled in my direction. "I no!"

Stunned and confused, I blinked. Moments earlier I had heard the twins singing outdoors. What on earth had happened? Would Maria forfeit her allowance because she was mad at her sister? Why? Or was this simply a sign that she felt safe enough in our home to let loose the moods that sometimes blew through her like a freight train? Did she resent our treating her like an American child by giving her an allowance?

The weekly allowance was intended to help the girls learn the value of money. Now, I realized we couldn't know what that American practice might convey to children from another culture.

Before I could gather my wits to speak, Maria whisked past me, marched to her bedroom, and slammed the door. I wished that I could crawl inside her head to understand her thoughts and feelings. She had no way of telling me. Quite likely, she didn't know herself.

It was one of many moments when I wished I had put more effort into learning to speak Russian. Mike and I had studied a book for beginners and received tutoring from

Ella, but the Cyrillic alphabet threw us for a loop. We had memorized a few sentences and a long list of vocabulary words, but never developed the skills to engage in a deep parent–child conversation.

Later, I was still feeling helpless and frazzled by the incident when Maria emerged from the bedroom and snuggled up beside me. "I sorry, Gail," she said remorsefully.

"For what?" I asked, hoping I might get some insight into what had caused her to fly off the handle.

"I bad," she said, summing up the incident.

"It's okay, Maria," I responded. "You were mad."

I never learned what had caused Maria's blowup. It was one of many conundrums I struggled with that summer regarding the complexities of parenting, language, money, gifting, personality, and culture.

Another day, two other girls from the Children of Chernobyl program came to our house to play with Maria and Vika. They arrived with portable audio players purchased by their host family. When I saw the twins' eyes grow wide with envy, I knew the stage was set for another lesson in consumerism and desire.

"Maybe I and Maria players?" Vika asked after the guests left.

Mike and I exchanged a silent acknowledgment of dread. Though we could afford to buy them, and we both liked to purchase gifts for the girls, we didn't want to set a precedent of keeping up with the neighbors. More importantly, we couldn't know how the twins' parents would view the situation.

"No," said Mike. His abrupt reaction sliced like a knife.

Vika blinked back tears. Maria slumped on the sofa. My eyes screamed at Mike, *How could you be so cruel?* Though in principle I agreed with him, I wanted to let them down gently.

"Zoya and Ivan would have to buy batteries constantly to keep them going," he reminded me. "They're expensive."

"You're right," I said. But Vika persisted.

"I need on *samolet*," Vika argued. On the *airplane*. "Then I no sick." She knew we didn't scrimp on health care and other essentials and wouldn't want her to suffer if she became ill on the long flight back to Moscow. But her creative strategy failed.

"I think you'll be okay on the plane," Mike laughed.

I knew a Walkman wouldn't improve her health, but I found myself wondering if I would buy a player for my own ten-year-old child. It seemed like every kid in America had one. Of course, that didn't mean it was a good idea to send Maria and Vika home with electronics. But, still feeling the pain of telling Vika she couldn't have the carved-leather journal, I couldn't seem to drop it.

"What if they used their allowance for half the cost?" I suggested. "I saw Walkmans on sale at Bartell Drugs for twenty dollars." Hope flashed in Vika's eyes. Maria perked up.

"What about the batteries?" Mike asked, now regarding me as a traitor. "They may not even be able to use the audio players in Zalessie."

"We could send a box of batteries home with them," I suggested, against my better judgment.

The girls sensed the tide had turned. Smugness changed the contour of their faces, and I realized I had passed the point of changing course. Even Mike knew it was over. He capitulated with a shrug of his shoulders. The girls ran to count their money. I wasn't sure I had conveyed the kind of message Mike and I had hoped for, but the girls did have to wait a week to collect another allowance before they could make their purchases.

Soon after they acquired the Walkmans, we made our second pilgrimage to Lake Chelan. Often, the girls bickered during long stretches in the car. On this trip across the state, however, they were unusually quiet. I checked to see if they'd fallen asleep. But they were wide awake, headphones plugged into their ears, heads bobbing to music.

"We should have bought those players sooner!" I joked.

As I enjoyed the quiet, my mind drifted back to the previous summer, when the girls sang our way home from Chelan through an old-growth forest. I knew I would regret giving them permission to buy the music players if they were too absorbed in private Walkman worlds, this year, to sing us home again.

CHAPTER 15

❖ Work and Play the Old World Way

My worries that Vika's and Maria's creativity would yield to battery-powered entertainment soon faded. Despite the Walkmans in our midst, America Number Three—as the girls referred to that summer—delivered a time of homespun pleasures and sharpened our awareness of cultural differences in entertainment.

The twins introduced us to laughing competitions, a game of good medicine for people of all ages. The winner is the one whose laugh induces the most laughter among all the other players.

Vika kicked off the competition by squealing and chortling like a flock of wild turkeys. Her facial contortions kept us all in stitches. By the time she ran out of steam, I had my arms wrapped around my sides to keep my ribs from hurting.

Maria stepped up as contestant number two. After a deep breath, she clutched her throat and launched into an ear-piercing cackle. Screeching, she threw back her head and rolled her eyeballs skyward until all that was visible were crooked red veins. I was bent in half, convulsing with laughter, when Maria ran out of breath and turned to me.

"Now you, Gail."

I drew a blank. The twins' acts were hard to follow. I felt self-conscious and couldn't imagine how to proceed. But something busted loose in me. I began laughing and, inadvertently, snorting like a pig. The ridiculous sounds shocked me as well as my audience. The surprise on Mike's and the twins' faces released my inner stand-up comic and spurred me on. I kept going until tears of laughter blurred my vision and I exhausted myself.

After Mike's Woody Woodpecker approach—*hahahaha-hahahaha*—which barely lifted the laughing meter, we took a vote. Maria's performance won hands down.

Another form of entertainment Vika and Maria introduced involved transforming Mike into Boris Yeltsin, then president of Russia. *What ten-year-old kids create look-alikes of foreign presidents?* I wondered. Most of the children I knew enjoyed dressing up as superheroes or princesses and other characters they saw on television and in movies; I doubted many of them could even *name* the prime minister of Canada or the president of Mexico, our neighbors to the north and south.

"But Yeltsin is old! And fat!" Mike protested. Giggling, the girls fussed with his hair and plumped his stomach with a pillow under his shirt.

"Yeltsin has a full head of hair. Mike, no hair," I commented.

"Just a minute," replied Maria, licking her fingers. We all burst into laughter when she glued Mike's thin strands of hair to his forehead with her saliva.

Finally satisfied with their Yeltsin project and ready to dive into something new, the girls lowered the blinds, lit candles, and treated the reluctant president and me to mesmerizing performances of gymnastics, ballet, and modern dance. Maria whirled gracefully and kicked with precision. Vika skillfully rolled and tumbled, and she played up her double-jointed versatility with a leg wrapped behind her neck. With no formal training, they delivered impressive skill and choreography that I knew reflected the government-controlled television programming in their home country. The only "superheroes" they saw on the screen were the stars of one-party politics in Belarus and Russia, Olympian heroes, and other performers who elevated a sense of national pride. A steady diet of classical Russian music, dance, athletics, and Yeltsin had produced the themes now playing out in my living room.

On another occasion, the girls introduced us to the lovely practice of reciting the names of friends and family members. *Yulia*, rhyming with Julia. *Doe-meen-ee-ka. Ar-seen-ee. Ba-rees.*

They sounded like two little monks chanting. I loved their ways of being inclusive, intimate, and present with Mike and me. It was the kind of emotional connection I had longed for as a child.

When Maria and Vika had named all their friends and kin from every generation they could remember, they asked to hear my family names.

Hazel. Clarence. Phyllis. Lester. . . . As I honored my elders by speaking their names, I received the unexpected gift of feeling a deep and satisfying connection to my roots. When I finished, Mike named his people. *Edna. Harold. Arlene. Ansel.* . . . Then we heard the names the twins might one day name their own children. *Alexsander. Anichka. Katryna. Valentyna. Nikita. Denys.* . . .

On another day, out of the blue, Vika suggested we clean the whole house together. "And rugs," she added. I gasped.

"Oh, Lord, help me!" I imagined chaos and collateral damage I couldn't allow.

"*I* help you," Vika corrected me.

I assumed this must have been a ritual Zoya and the girls performed in their one-bedroom apartment, or an annual spring cleaning they did for Babushka in Ukraine. Though her suggestion warmed my heart, I imagined my living room rug being dragged across the flower beds outside, the vacuum cleaner zooming toward my china cabinet, moving furniture that would leave scratches on the wood floors, and the beautiful figurine from Zoya smashed into smithereens.

"Maybe you like to wash the car instead?" I knew she couldn't say no to water.

The girls' eyes lit up. Without a word, they raced to their bedroom and changed into bathing suits. Tickled that my strategy had worked, I gathered sponges, filled a bucket with soapy water, and uncoiled the hose. While the girls washed and rinsed the car, I relaxed on the deck, enjoying their happy chatter, birds chirping, and bamboo rustling in the breeze.

As summer drew to a close, we were in the car one day when the girls observed a group of teenagers standing beside the road waving signs and calling to drivers.

"What, Gail?" Vika asked, wondering what the kids were up to.

"They are washing cars to make money for their soccer team," I explained. "Maybe so they can buy new soccer clothes."

"*Chto?*" Maria asked, turning to Vika. *What?*

Vika explained in Russian, and the subject was dropped. But the next time we stopped at a gas station, the girls hopped out of the car with Mike. Familiar with his ritual of cleaning the windows while the tank was filling, they offered to clean the windows for 50 cents. When he agreed, they went to work. Peering in at me through the glass, they were all smiles. Vika's USA T-shirt stretched across her chest as she strained to reach the middle of the windshield.

While Maria and Vika gleefully sprayed and squeegeed the windows, I thought about the joys these two remarkable girls had cooked up for Mike and me, using only what they had absorbed from their culture. The dopamine-inducing laughing game. Names recited like prayer mantras. Talents inspired by Russian gymnasts and dancers. Songs sung by their family while their papa played an accordion.

As I marveled at the mystery and good fortune of creating family with these two particular girls, Mike tapped on the window, startling me.

"Gailey," he called, using an endearment I loved.

"Yeah?"

"How do the windows look?" The girls stood by him, awaiting my assessment.

I angled my head, checking for smears. "Good!" I concluded.

"Did the girls miss any spots? Did they do a good job?" He was laying it on heavy for our two entrepreneurs.

"Crystal clear!"

"Okay! Good job, girls!" he said, handing them each a quarter.

Back on the highway, the girls conversed in the back seat like two businesswomen creating a start-up. I turned to Mike.

"Zoya and Ivan won't be happy if the girls are capitalists when they come home," I said, laughing uneasily.

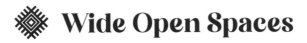 **Wide Open Spaces**

My friend Jennifer burst into the house like a whirlwind, a PERFUME POLLUTES button pinned to her jacket and scarves dangling from her neck.

"Talent show! MCS picnic. We're singing with Vika and Maria!" Her brown eyes sparkled with a vision of performing at the annual summer gathering of our MCS support group.

I admired my spitfire friend's courage, creativity, and spunk in matters of the heart—both personal and political. To function in her workplace, where she'd been made deathly ill from chemical toxins during an office renovation, she now had to wear a respirator to avoid landing in the hospital from a reaction to fragrances. And she needed to wear it to attend performances at Seattle's Fifth Avenue Theatre, where she had purchased season tickets. I might have stayed home rather than sit in a theatre wearing a gas mask. But not Jennifer. With heavy-duty canisters covering her nose and mouth, she showed up early and stood outside, under the marquee lights, wearing a sexy black dress and high heels, handing out pamphlets on the dangers of fragrances to ticket holders as they arrived. She was a natural performer and storyteller, a song and dance girl.

For me, the thought of performing on stage evoked a determined resistance. "Not going to happen, Jenn," I informed her. "You know I can't sing."

"Sure you can!" she insisted. "I've got the perfect song: 'Wide Open Spaces' by the Dixie Chicks."

"I've never even heard of the Dixie Chicks," I confessed.

"They're an all-girl country music band from Texas," she explained. "'Wide Open Spaces' is about women's independence, and it's making them super popular right now."

Seated on a sage and coral Persian rug, Maria and Vika listened intently to our banter, trying to decipher what the excitement was all about. Their eyes ricocheted between Jennifer and me.

"All you have to do is learn the lyrics. I'll do the costumes and choreography." As usual, Jennifer wouldn't take no for an answer. Despite my aversion, her enthusiasm began to rub off on me.

"It does sound like fun," I admitted. "And the MCS group *is* easy to please. They'd appreciate anyone brave enough to get up on the stage."

Jenn swung her long salt-and-pepper hair from side to side and pumped her arm above her head. "Yessss!"

The twins understood we'd hatched a plan but had no clue what it entailed. "Gail, *chto*? *Chto?*" Vika asked urgently. *What?*

"You, me, Jennifer," I said, pointing to each of us, "sing and dance for many people," I tried to explain. The girls got my drift immediately. Squealing like two passengers set for takeoff on a magic carpet, they flew to their feet and danced.

Over the next three weeks, every time we rode in the car, one of us popped in the Dixie Chicks cassette and turned up the volume. Up one Seattle hill and down another, we practiced singing our song—about leaving home, chasing dreams, and heading west—on our way to the pool, the library, the market, and home again.

Though the twins didn't fully understand the meaning of the lyrics, the song was a perfect fit for two Belarusian girls who'd found a second home in America. The words also struck home for me, a woman called by ocean and mountains to create a life in the American West, far removed from roots and family; a woman whose dreams had been derailed by environmental illness and infertility.

We sang and practiced the choreography with Jennifer until we could sidestep and shake our tail feathers to the beat with sass. As a former member of the US synchronized swim team, Jenn knew how to impress an audience, and she delivered.

On the evening of the talent show, our group of thirty adults and a gaggle of children gathered in a large picnic shelter at the Good Shepherd Center, a historical landmark built in 1906 as a home for two hundred nuns and way-ward girls. Sitting on eleven acres, surrounded by a winding rock wall, a playground, and organic gardens, it provided a perfect oasis for our group of refugees from industrialized America. No one wore fragranced personal care products or clothing laundered with scented detergent or fabric soft-ener. No pesticides were used to maintain the grounds. The environment enabled us to socialize without feeling ill or suffering consequences to our health. And, because food sensitivities are also problematic for many people who suffer from reactions to fragrances and other chemicals, the foods we brought to share were all gluten- and dairy-free, and each dish came with a list of ingredients.

Vika and Maria took to the party atmosphere with exuberance. Perhaps they also resonated with a familiar ambiance, something they couldn't have named but felt in the MCS group—a gaiety that asserts itself when the grief of a diminished life is temporarily forgotten. Chemicals and radiation had given us that in common.

The freedom to socialize without fear of becoming ill from exposures intoxicated me. For the first time, the girls saw me gadding about and hugging people without reservation. They were accustomed to the accommodations my life normally required—avoiding crowds, declining hugs from people outside my safe inner circle, leaving restaurants before I'd finished eating when fragrances or gas stove fumes drifted my way.

"Start the show!" someone called, eager for the entertainment to begin after we'd finished eating.

We all arranged ourselves on chairs and tabletops, facing the lawn. Two women wearing silly wigs got the ball rolling with a duet. Strumming guitars and singing a comical song they'd written about living with MCS, they soon had everyone in stitches. A string of performances followed: a child playing a flute, a woman singing a cappella, a magic act.

As our turn to perform drew near, Jennifer, the twins, and I stood by a garden of towering sunflowers, cascading amaranth, and herbs, waiting for our cue. Just as our song began to play, a wave of jitters hit me. *What had I been thinking?*

Maria drummed her chest and cleared her throat. Vika's blue-green eyes flashed with the thrill of stardom. I took a deep breath and caught the calming scent of basil floating from the garden.

"Smile!" Jennifer reminded us.

With bandanas tied around our necks and suede-fringed earrings swinging just above our shoulders, the four of us boogied out onto the lawn strumming imaginary guitars. Standing in pairs at center stage, Jennifer and Vika locked eyes, flirting as they sang together; Maria and I wagged our heads close to each other's, singing and strumming. A wild spark lit Maria's willow-green eyes in the evening glow. We do-si-doed and switched partners. Vika then fixed her bewitching eyes on me, and we locked arms. Her strong, tanned arm held me tight. The crowd cheered.

With every beat, the pulse of a powerful current grew within and between us, grounding and resonant. I realized it was the feminine energy that arises when we own what is ours to risk, to heal, to grow.

During an instrumental midway through our performance, our country western number took on a new dimension. Keeping time with the music, Jennifer and I moved to the side. The twins stepped forward to wow the audience with an acrobatic duet they had choreographed themselves. They twisted, flipped, and rolled to the delight of a cheering audience. Applause erupted when Vika executed her startling, double-jointed maneuver, placing one leg against the back of her head. Right on time, we regrouped to launch into the final chorus.

That night when the girls climbed into bed, we were still pulsing with the elixir of applause and claiming our voices. When I bent down to kiss Vika good night, she grabbed my cheeks and pulled my face so close to hers that my eyes crossed.

"Gail, I'm *so proud* of you!" she crowed.

At first, I was stunned. *When did she learn to say that in English?* Then I blushed, and a giddy delight splashed over me like a warm wave. Feeling truly seen in a new way by the ten-year-old girl holding my face, I knew this was a moment I would savor for a lifetime.

Vika understood that I had stepped beyond my comfort zone and claimed more of my own power that night. Together we had created something akin to the beauty and glory of candles burning brightly and melting together. Though she was thrilled by the response to her own star turn, she was equally pleased by my success.

Immersed in the indescribable glow of motherhood, I whispered, "Good night" when she finally released me.

Part Five:
2001

CHAPTER 17

🔷 The Unspeakable Fusion of Light and Loss

Just three months shy of their thirteenth birthday, the twins had already morphed into teenagers by the time they sashayed into Seattle for our summer 2001 reunion. Vika had the curves of a young woman beginning to take shape; her eyes glowed with a warm presence. Maria stood tall, her hair cut short with gentle waves framing her face, her sea-green eyes still bright with a touch of fiery amber.

"You girls have grown up!" I trilled, stroking Vika's thick, shiny mane draped over her back and shoulders like a caramel-colored veil.

It had been two years since our last visit. Reeling from the death of Mike's brother in 2000, Mike and I had been unable to host Maria and Vika that summer. This would be their fourth and final trip with the Children of Chernobyl. The girls were aging out of the program.

To make up for lost time, both past and future, Mike and I had planned two memory-making trips with the twins—one to Lake Chelan with Mike's sister and her children, and one to Michigan.

Not yet knowing how fate would soon disappoint us, we kicked off America Number Four at a housewarming party for Alex and Ella at their new three-bedroom home near Lake Washington. The party was in full swing when we arrived from the airport. We removed our shoes at the door and stepped onto a striking white sheepskin rug, pausing to acclimate. Scents of chicken, cabbage, and roses perfumed the room. Buzzing with laughter and vodka, a group of Ukrainian and Russian immigrants, seated shoulder to shoulder around a long oval table draped in white damask, lifted their shot glasses to welcome us. Alex squeezed four more chairs up to the table for us.

At the center stood a large bouquet of long-stemmed red roses set in a crystal vase, surrounded by platters of chicken cutlets, salami, smoked fish, cabbage rolls, vodka, dill pickle chasers, and boxes of Russian chocolates. A sea of salads mixed with mayonnaise covered the remainder of the tabletop: Finely chopped mushrooms and garlic with black pepper. Imitation crab with rice and corn. Diced potatoes, carrots, eggs, and peas. Grated beets. Cauliflower florets with garlic and cheese.

Vika and Maria participated in the banter as though they'd known these strangers forever. Though Mike and I were outsiders—the only non-Russian speakers—our relationship with Alex and Ella and the twins allowed us a comfortable sense of belonging amid the chaos and conversation we didn't understand. Whenever possible, we used a Russian word or two. *Da. Pozhaluysta. Spacibo.*

When the feasting slowed, Ella passed around the chocolates and urged the twins to sing for us. *"Pozhaluysta!"* everyone pleaded. *Please!* To our delight, the twins agreed.

With infinitesimal bits of native earth and air still clinging to their shoes, their skin, their breath, they perfumed the room with an intoxicating elixir. Blushing in the spotlight, Maria touched the audience with her soprano voice. Vika held them in the gaze of her mandala eyes. The old-world tone of their voices called the soul of Ukraine into this Seattle house.

Transported back to their villages, Ella and her guests fixed their eyes on the twins of innocence. They roared with enthusiasm and applause.

The girls' tone and tempo changed dramatically with their second number, a somber piece. Ella and some of her women friends started to cry softly. The men dabbed their eyes with the backs of their hands. The heavy weight of a haunted place sucked air from the room.

Though I couldn't understand the lyrics, the lament ushered me back to the day of Mike's brother's death in the bedroom he and Mike had shared as children in their parents' house. Weak and frail, his eyes were closed and he appeared to be sleeping when I went in the room to check on him. But to my surprise, I heard him speak.

"Tell them I'll see them tonight."

Was he talking to someone in the spirit world? I hoped he was conversing with his beloved Grandma Friebe, whose Sunday dinners and lively card parties remained the talk of the town long after her life had ended. Jeff, a former teacher and mayor of a village in southwest Michigan, loved parties and conversation. He loved to share stories about his experiences in the navy aboard a submarine, most likely the source of his exposure to asbestos.

Peacefulness permeated the room and held me there. Jeff said nothing more. The clock ticking on the wall in the hallway made the only sound. I wanted to remain present to every nuance of grace that opened death's door, as I had been unable to do as a teenager when my beloved brother, Jim, died of melanoma at the age of twenty-one.

Jim was my hero, the man I looked up to even more than I did to my father. When he was dying, I had been too devastated and needy to say goodbye. Unable to imagine finding my way in a world without him, I couldn't bear to see the light fading in his eyes. But I was learning that every moment is sacred as the end of a life approaches. This time I would not turn away.

When Jeff took his final breath, Mike, his parents, and I were standing at his bedside. My body swayed forward and back, and side to side, as waves of pain and gratitude swelled and broke. That sea suddenly calmed, and the separation between grief and gratitude no longer existed. There was only love. I felt thankful to be present for that transcendent moment.

Now, at Ella's, listening to the girls sing, that holy state revisited me, the oneness of grief and gratitude, the essence of love. I didn't understand how I had entered that state until Ella explained, after the song ended, "They sing about Chernobyl. Tell about how everything in homeland turned black, everything die. They see terrible truth of conditions in Belarus and Ukraine. Not see with child's eyes." Tears still welled in Ella's eyes. She gestured to her friends seated around the table. "Make us miss Ukraine," she added, "and grateful we now live in United States."

Pain and loss create portals to love. That terrible truth had brought Maria and Vika into my life and changed the geography of my interior landscape. That paradox had birthed the global family that was healing my wounds.

The mood in the room lifted when the girls launched into a witty tune that made people laugh and then ended with a love song. We left the party on a high note and headed home to engage in our gifting ritual and to unpack the familiar black duffel. Visions of the weeks ahead danced in my head. I was especially eager to introduce our twins—and the parts of me they brought out—to my mother and sister and nieces and nephew in Michigan.

At home, Maria pulled from their bag two small Mother Mary icons in carved wood frames, one with Mary alone and one with baby Jesus cradled in her arms. "From Babushka," she said, handing them to me.

"So you won't be sad when I and Maria leave," explained Vika.

Touching the pictures, I imagined Babushka in a shadowed room scented with grief and dill, removing the icons from a wall to send to Mike and me. We'd never met, yet I could feel her caring presence. Though I didn't know it yet, she was a survivor of famine, a world war, the Chernobyl explosion, and the early death of her beloved husband.

Perhaps Babushka sensed that grief was on its way to pay me a visit.

CHAPTER 18

◈ Brainstorms and Blessings

A terrifying downward spiral announced itself late one evening when a strange sensation grabbed hold of me. In my own home, surrounded by familiar objects infused with love and cherished memories, I suddenly felt severed from emotion and meaning. Nothing in the room had changed. A switch in my brain had flipped.

I gazed at the twins' shoes sitting by the door, the cabinet filled with china I had inherited from my mother, the oil lamp my grandparents had used to light their farmhouse. Though I knew the stories attached to everything in the room, those stories were no longer connected to my heartstrings. I felt like an untethered soul held hostage by a distorted reality. Panic reverberated through me from head to toe.

I turned to Mike in alarm. "Something's wrong."

"What do you mean?"

"I don't feel right." Worry crept over his eyes. "Everything seems strange," I tried to explain. "Even you and the girls. I feel like I don't have a self."

"Maybe you're just tired," he said, taking me into his arms. "It's late. Let's go to bed. Maybe sleep will help."

Neither of us made the connection, then, between this frightening experience and my car accident two months earlier.

While driving alone not far from home, I'd been struck head-on by a vehicle traveling the wrong direction in my lane. Neither I nor the other driver could see the crash coming until moments before we collided at the top of a rise in the road. For weeks I suffered from debilitating head pain and muscle spasms. With the help of acupuncture and massage, those symptoms had subsided by the time of the twins' July arrival. But I had still been experiencing quick flashes of something that felt like doom, fuzzy pieces of nightmares on the edges of my peripheral vision. I had chalked those up to temporary remnants of the accident and felt confident that the girls' presence would soon clear those trauma echoes out of my nervous system.

Now I lay awake like a zombie. Anxiety cut through me like a razor. It took hours before I finally drifted into sleep. When I first woke in the morning, I felt miraculously normal again, reconnected to myself and safe in the world. The ability to *feel* the simple pleasure of hearing the morning chatter of chickadees floating through the open window flooded me with relief. Still, I called my acupuncturist and scheduled an appointment.

That afternoon, Vika and Maria watched in fascination as the old doctor, a bamboo-thin Chinese man, stuck needles into my arms, legs, and head. After he had finished and left the room, the girls sang to me while the needles worked their magic. The twins' presence, their voices, and the blending of Chinese medicine with Belarusian music filled the treatment room with joyful, healing pulses that left me feeling ecstatic.

The next day I took the girls to their happy place—the community pool. I, too, was in my element in water, especially when swimming with my girls. But my condition deteriorated after that outing.

By the next morning, I couldn't care for myself or cope with normal everyday life. Sounds caused unbearable suffering. The ringing of a phone shook me like an earthquake. We had to silence our phones and television. Even the sound of a normal conversation between others in the same room rocked my nervous system. My vision seemed split, as if my left and right eyes weren't in sync. I lay on the sofa too weak to even eat.

The only explanation Mike and I could think of was brain damage caused by the auto accident. But why hadn't the damage been evident earlier? We didn't yet realize that turning my head repetitively and stretching my neck up out of the water had exacerbated the effects of the whiplash I had sustained in the collision.

Watching my life spark disappear, and with his brother's death still fresh in his memory, Mike flew into action. He arranged for Maria and Vika to stay with Ella for a few days while we dealt with my health crisis, and he made an appointment for me to see a neurologist.

An MRI showed no abnormalities. "There's nothing wrong with you that antidepressants can't fix," the neurologist claimed. But this was nothing like the depression I'd ever experienced myself or witnessed as a mental health professional.

Desperate for help, I called a brain injury organization. The volunteer who answered my call informed me that I was experiencing classic symptoms of MTBI—mild traumatic brain injury—which interferes with brain function but isn't visible on diagnostic scans. In a conversation with someone who had experienced MTBI, I was encouraged to consult with a local doctor known for his expertise in upper cervical alignment, a specialized form of chiropractic treatment focused on the brain-body connection.

The following day, that doctor examined me, took measurements and X-rays, and offered a possible explanation for my sudden, mysterious symptoms. My atlas—the top vertebra of the spinal column, connecting the skull and spine—was misaligned, he explained, creating pressure on my brain stem. He felt confident the realignment of my atlas would help and cautioned me that it could take months for it to hold. The treatment began that day.

As I lay on my side on the exam table, my head resting awkwardly on a slightly raised platform, the doctor stood over me and gently placed the edge of his hand just below my ear. There was no twisting of my head or neck. In fact, he barely touched me.

"There! Good," he said. The maneuver had taken no more than thirty seconds, and I had felt almost nothing. Over time this treatment would make a significant improvement in my health—including my tolerance for chemical exposures and depression—but the results were gradual.

It soon became clear to Mike and me that I couldn't make the trip we had planned to Lake Chelan with his sister and her children. I couldn't even carry on a conversation. My disappointment was surpassed only by how badly I felt for disappointing the twins. It was not possible to explain to them what was happening to me. We simplified by telling them my head hurt terribly. The truth was that the impingement on my brain stem had blown a fuse in my nervous system.

"Bad for you. Bad for me," Vika said.

Ideally, Mike would have gone to Chelan with the rest of the gang, which would have minimized the impact on him and the others. But he was unwilling to leave me alone, and, in my compromised condition, I felt afraid to stay home without him. Instead, friends of ours canceled their own family vacation plans to take our place. They met Mike's sister, her children, and the twins in Chelan so Debbie wouldn't be there on her own with five children for the week.

Hell-bent on improving my health while the girls were gone, I did everything in my power to rebuild my strength and equilibrium. Following a regimen of atlas adjustments, acupuncture, medications, psychotherapy, nutritional supplements, naps, meditation, prayer, and nature walks, I vowed I would come through the setback stronger than I had been before the accident.

When Debbie and the five children returned, I still felt fragile but strong enough to have them all spend a night with us. When they arrived, I burst into tears, partly because I was so happy to see them and partly because I realized how much I had missed. I knew those feelings were mutual when, every time I sat down, one of the girls squeezed into the chair with me.

With that physical connection, and their stories of swimming, jet skis, snow cones, and *Ozero* Chelan flying around the room, my world felt right again. But my heart broke once more when I faced the fact that I still didn't have the stamina to travel with the girls to Michigan as planned. Mike's parents had met them during their first summer visit, when we hosted a Friebe family reunion in Seattle. But my family would never see and experience me as a mother or fall under Vika and Maria's spell. To them, my twins would always be a story, not an unforgettable firsthand encounter with their spontaneity, bravery, affection, giggles, dancing, and singing. We would not create memories together that would leave traces of my girls in their homes and hearts. They would not see, firsthand, the bridge I had built or the dream I'd brought to life out of the ashes of infertility. The twins would never step foot on the land where that dream had first taken shape during the Cold War. And we would never have another chance to connect the girls to our roots.

Fortunately, the full range of those losses didn't hit me all at once. Over time I realized, bit by painful bit, just how much I had emotionally invested in that trip.

As if that weren't enough disappointment, my precarious condition meant that we still couldn't keep the girls with us full time. As a last resort, if we didn't come up with an alternative, Mike would have to escort the girls back to Moscow four weeks early.

Fortunately, friends came to our rescue again. Alex and Ella agreed to keep the twins with them during the week and shuffle them back to our house for the weekends. We enrolled them in a Russian gymnastics camp, where Alex dropped them off each morning, Monday through Friday, to keep them engaged and supervised while he and Ella worked.

As much as Vika and Maria loved Ella and Alex, the forced separation from us had the unexpected impact of kindling their longings for Mike and me. Vika called every evening to ask the same questions.

"How you feel, Gail? Maybe we come home tomorrow? *Russkiy* camp not so very good." I must admit that, after three summers of their protests whenever I picked them up from Ella's, Vika's aching to "come home" melted my heart.

Reminiscing, storytelling, and Vika's hilarious impersonations kept us happily entertained for hours in quiet scenic spots on our weekends with the girls. Sitting beside the Lake Washington Ship Canal one day, watching boats streaming by, Vika delivered an impersonation of Mike trying to get Maria to eat vegetables on previous visits.

"'Maria no eat two green beans, no *marozhina*!'" She spoke in a deep, husky voice that made even Maria laugh.

"Remember Vika make Yeltsin?" Maria asked. "Is very good, I think."

"Oh yes! Very good," I agreed, recalling the fun we had one summer when Vika, slurring her words and walking like a drunken sailor, had impersonated Boris Yeltsin, then president of Russia. "And when you girls turned Mike into Yeltsin, that very good, too!"

As we passed the hours with intentional slowness and simplicity, I realized we were capturing a special sweetness we might otherwise have missed in the hustle and bustle of normal life. Instead of packing in extra activities, we were stringing together memories of their four summer sojourns like beads on an heirloom necklace. We were deepening the bonds that I hoped would outlive Maria and Vika's participation in the Children of Chernobyl group and Mike's and my roles as volunteers.

After three weeks of camp, the twins came "home" to spend their final week in the United States with us. During that last week, we boarded a ferry to Bremerton, the same giant green-and-white vessel Mike and I had taken the day of the Chernobyl explosion. It was another beautiful day on Puget Sound, a section of the legendary Ring of Fire that included part of Siberia. A circle was closing. Soon the girls would return to Belarus, never to return with the Children of Chernobyl group.

Standing on the upper deck near the bridge, we four startled to the blast of the horn as the mammoth vessel pulled away from the dock. Seagulls swirled and squealed in the breeze. Cormorants raised their wet wings to dry them in the sun. We counted jellyfish floating in the water and watched for orcas, hoping to catch a glimpse of the Salish Sea's beloved killer whales.

My thoughts began to drift. *Where do we go from here?* I wondered. I was trying to picture my future without the girls' summer visits when Vika suddenly shrieked.

"Look! Look!" She was pointing to the ferry's port side.

"A giant moon jellyfish!" I cried. The gauzy, fringed, undulating disc was lit with a flower-shaped bulb embedded inside. Its trailing tentacles propelled it forward, extending and contracting with the reach and grace of a Bolshoi Ballet dancer.

"Ohmigod!" Maria exclaimed.

The girls' rapture and the exquisite beauty of the maritime dancer reminded me to let go of worries about the future and trust that mystery would carry me forward, moment by present moment.

As with each previous summer, the day before they were to leave, the girls grew restless, eager to reunite with their mama and papa and sister. While Mike supervised the packing, I slipped out to the store where, two years earlier, Vika had fallen in love with a journal bound with carved leather. She had been too young, then, to understand its purpose. But now it seemed like a perfect gift for her and Maria's thirteenth birthday. Luckily, the store still carried the beautiful books, and I purchased one for each girl. When I returned carrying a bag, the twins insisted I show them my purchase.

"It's a surprise for your birthday," I said, closing the bedroom door behind me. "Stay out."

Both girls dropped to the floor, trying to peek through the crack beneath the door. Not knowing how much longer they could restrain themselves, I hastily wrapped their gifts in pink and purple flowered paper, with both journals in a single box to throw the junior detectives off track. When I emerged with the package, trimmed with purple ribbons and shiny Mardi Gras beads, Maria and Vika jumped to their feet, poised to tear the paper to shreds.

"You can't open it until your birthday," I said, holding the tantalizing box over my head.

"I no wait! I open in Zalessie," threatened Vika.

"No, Mama won't let you open it until your birthday," I assured her. Though we were on separate continents, Zoya and I had each other's backs.

"Gail, no wait," Maria pleaded in her dejected hound dog voice.

While I distracted the girls with plans for the evening, Mike buried the gift in a giant duffel they had filled along with their little bag. We had purchased the oversized duffel at the navy surplus store, as we had done each previous visit, to hold everything the girls had accumulated over the summer and would take back to Zalessie.

"After dinner, we go to Taizé," I announced. I wanted to share a quiet and meaningful evening with the girls on their last night. With no idea when or if we would be together again, I hoped a holy experience would seal the bond between us with an indestructible mystical power.

Taizé was something we'd never talked about or done before, and I knew it would capture their curiosity. When I tried to explain, the twins gawked at me in confusion.

"*Chto?*" Vika asked.

"We go to church," I answered.

I didn't know enough Russian words to convey that Taizé was a nondenominational prayer service for people of any faith, language, or culture. I certainly couldn't have explained that it began in France, after World War II, to bring together prisoners, orphans, and refugees of warring countries, in a healing environment of peace and Spirit.

Vika scrunched her face into a scowl. "Church?"

"Yes, but no sermon. Nobody talks. We'll sit in silence part of the time and sing chants part of the time. There is music and candlelight. I think you'll like it." Though Vika was still skeptical, she didn't protest, and to my surprise, neither did Maria.

Beams of purple, red, and golden light shot through stained-glass niches behind the pulpit as we entered the sanctuary. Candlelight shadowed the walls as we slid into a pew near the back. Hidden behind a screen, the choir began singing a chant.

"*Holy Spirit, come to me. Holy Spirit, come to me . . .*"

With firelight dancing in their eyes, the twins joined Mike and me in singing.

I was a seeker of Spirit, but not a religious person. Drawn to interfaith practices, ancient stone circles in the fields of Scotland, and the feminine spirit of God, I believed in prayer. Though I wasn't a Catholic, I often prayed to Mother Mary.

A queue formed in the aisle for those of us who chose to light a candle and pray in silence at the altar. When I rose to take a place in line, Vika and Maria both followed, hands clasped on their tummies, a soft, buttery glow illuminating their faces.

Slowly, we approached a constellation of burning tapers standing in a tray of sand. When our turn came, we each picked up an unlit candle and tilted them toward a single flame. Our tapers burst to life simultaneously, like a guiding star. We planted them in the sand, in a galaxy of lighted prayers.

Holiness wrapped its arms around me as I stood beside my girls. Surrendering to grace, I prayed for their health and happiness, and the longevity of both our bridge and family. When I left the altar, returning to my place beside Mike, the girls' eyes were closed. I hoped their prayers would be answered. Soon, as if floating on a river of mystery and love, they slipped back in between us.

Later that night we stood outside in our pajamas gazing into the night sky where a big orange slice of moon hung over Puget Sound.

"*Krasivaya luna*," said Vika dreamily.

"*Da*. Beautiful moon," I agreed. It was the one thing we would still share when we were separated by ocean, earth, and air. Knowing we would always view the same moon provided me with the comfort of a touchstone I could never lose. In the months and years to come, I would understand that, like the moon, our relationship would wax and wane over time.

 # 9/11

Three weeks after saying goodbye to the twins, our phone rang early one morning. Mike was packing for a business trip. Awake but still in bed, I glanced at the caller ID. It was my niece Tammy in Michigan. My heart immediately began to race. At that hour, only bad news could be the reason for her call. Bracing myself, I picked up the phone.

"Where's Mike?" She knew he traveled frequently for work. The alarm in her voice shook me. *Oh God, something unthinkable has happened in our family. She knows I'm going to need Mike.*

"Getting ready to go to the airport. What's wrong?" I began to feel light-headed and disoriented.

"Tell him not to go! Terrorists hijacked a plane and crashed into the World Trade Center in New York. They think other flights have been hijacked. Turn on your television!"

It was September 11, 2001. Adrenaline, confusion, and fear ran through me in circles. The United States was under attack.

As Mike and I watched on television, a hijacked airliner struck the second tower of the World Trade Center and a third airliner crashed into the Pentagon.

My emotions cycled between terrified and numb. *Is this the beginning of World War III? Will I ever see my family again? Thank God Vika and Maria weren't on one of those flights!* To my amazement, Mike left the room, collected his bag and briefcase, and headed toward the door.

"You're not leaving!" I insisted.

"I have to catch my flight," he snapped. Apparently in shock, he was acting like a robot programmed to work even as a national crisis was unfolding.

"Are you out of your mind? Every flight in the US has been grounded. It was just announced." Allowing that reality to sink in, he stopped, put away his bags, and sat.

We watched in disbelief and horror as, over the next thirty minutes, the 110-story Twin Towers of the World Trade Center collapsed, and another hijacked airliner crashed in Pennsylvania. As videos of the disasters replayed over and over, I asked myself, *What good have I done by spending years building a bridge of peace?* The notion that a human bridge could counter this scourge now struck me as naive.

When I couldn't stand to watch another replay of the World Trade Center collapsing, I decided to take a walk. I needed to feel what I couldn't yet grasp. New York was thousands of miles away. Here, on the West Coast, there was no visible proof of the damage. Still, the world as I knew it would never be the same.

As I walked up the hill outside my house, my heart began to pound from exertion, fear, or both. *Take it easy. You're okay. Breathe.* I tried to ground and soothe myself by staying focused on the beauty surrounding me. A garden of purple sedums. A clear blue sky. Gold mums. Puget Sound glittering.

The autumn day couldn't have appeared more peaceful. Still, my eyes darted left to right, expecting an armed man to ambush me at any moment. As a female, I was accustomed to feeling vulnerable and taking precautions to protect myself from danger, especially at night, but I had never felt unsafe in my own neighborhood, in the daylight. Now, I felt like a target, hated for being a US citizen.

Standing alone on Sunset Hill overlooking Puget Sound, trying to metabolize the horrible truth, I was struck by the absence of sounds. The usual parade of airliners going into and out of SeaTac Airport, cruising at low altitudes over the area, had been grounded. There were no cars or trucks speeding by. The city had gone mute, as if the world had stopped its frantic spinning. The moment felt both eerie and tinged with grace. *Remember this*, I told myself. *You may never hear the sound of stillness here again.*

A chorus of birdsong started. With no urban soundtrack playing in the background, the melody was clear and amplified, like bells ringing in a temple. Serene and bittersweet, the music evoked my tears of grief. With the Olympic Mountains as my only witness, I began to cry.

I couldn't yet know how our lives might be changed by this event, but because the 9/11 terrorists claimed to be Muslim, I knew that Islam would replace Russia as the face of evil in the United States. And I knew that I would not give up on my bridge.

Part Six:

2007

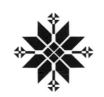

CHAPTER 20

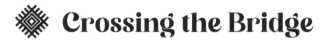 # Crossing the Bridge

Seattle to Ukraine

"Come with us!" pleaded Ella. Her dark eyes sparkled, and candlelight danced on the crystal wine goblet cupped in her hand.

We were celebrating Winter Solstice 2006 with a salmon dinner at my house. Ella and Alex had just announced they were planning their first trip back to Ukraine since emigrating twelve years earlier.

"First, I will go with you to Belarus, then we will take the train back to Ukraine to meet Alex in Vinnytsia. You'll see where we lived," Ella proposed. Her invitation struck me like the answered prayer I had both longed for and feared.

My desire to visit the twins in Belarus had all but consumed me for more than five years. I longed to see them again and to fully realize my childhood dream. As a host parent for the Children of Chernobyl program, I had already begun building a bridge. But I knew it wouldn't be complete until I immersed myself in Vika and Maria's culture. They had mustered the courage to cross that bridge as young children, and now it was my turn. But fear had stood in my way.

Ukraine didn't frighten me. There, a democracy was taking shape with freedom of speech and presidential elections scrutinized for corruption. Belarus, however, had maintained strong ties to Russia and disdain for the West. I'd read that the media was censored, and criticism of the government was punishable by law. The thought of entering President Alexander Lukashenko's domain terrified me.

The source of that fear was no mystery to me, a child of the Cold War raised on a diet of fear. Still, it wasn't as if I were someone who always played it safe or never left the country. I loved to explore different cultures and had traveled off the beaten path in Mexico, the Greek Islands, and northern Europe. I had uprooted myself from the Midwest and followed my heart to the Pacific Northwest, a place I'd never seen, where I didn't know a soul. But I'd never been in a country where free speech was not allowed.

"Come!" Ella repeated. Her enthusiasm charged the air.

I knew I would feel safe in Belarus with Ella, a native of Soviet culture and fluent in Russian, Ukrainian, and English. And I didn't want to miss the opportunity to accompany her and Alex to their hometowns, as a witness to their former lives in Ukraine. But I hadn't expected her generous offer, knowing it would cut her time with her own friends and family. It was a sacrifice I wouldn't have asked her to make.

"Really? You'd go to Belarus with us?"

"Of course. Come! My friends in Ukraine will be in shock when I come with American friends."

A flutter of excitement rose in my chest. A blur of thoughts and feelings tumbled through me. Mike's bushy eyebrows rose into question marks as he and our friends waited for my response.

"Let's do it!" I blurted. Everyone cheered.

Alex wasted no time arranging our June 2007 flights to Boryspil International Airport and renting an apartment in

Kyiv. After two nights in the capital city, he would travel to Vinnytsia to visit family and wait for us while Ella took a train to Belarus with Mike and me.

Day by day my excitement grew—until I started reading guidebooks that scared the bejesus out of me.

"Did you know you can go to jail in Belarus for taking pictures of government buildings?" I asked Mike.

"Uh-huh," he mumbled. Unfazed, he continued reading the newspaper.

"It says here, we have to check in at a government office to get a special stamp after we've been in Belarus for three days, or we won't be allowed to leave the country. Oh no! It also says some people are detained even when they've followed all the protocols!" My stomach twisted into knots.

"That's not going to happen," replied Mike flatly. He was a guy who wouldn't worry about finding enough water on a trek across a desert. I admired his optimism, but sometimes it went too far, crossing into a form of denial that helped him to cope with the unknown. This was one of those times when I wanted to shake him awake to the dark side of life. His lack of concern made me feel angry and alone.

"How do you know?" I exploded. "Everything I've read about Lukashenko describes him as an unscrupulous dictator. People who run against him *disappear* or land in *jail!*"

"That may be true, Gail, but you're not running for president of Belarus," he replied.

He had a point there, I had to admit, but my anxiety wouldn't subside. Though everyone I talked to reassured me that I'd be safe, ghosts of the Cold War haunted me night and day. I was convinced that even Ella's perspective had been skewed by years of Soviet brainwashing.

I thought about my mother with her guns and cringed. Was I becoming one of those people who automatically avoids or reacts with fear to people, places, and ideas outside their comfort zones? Years later, when I shared my story with a Russian woman I met in Hawaii, she validated my fears. "Of course you were afraid," she said. "You're used to having the protection of the law."

I remained determined to parse out truth from propaganda. Finally, when I was on the verge of telling Mike he would have to make the trip to Belarus without me, I contacted the author of one of the travel books I'd been reading, an American experienced in navigating Belarusian bureaucracy. When *he* assured me that—unless my name appeared on a blacklist of known political activists—I would be safe, a deep peace washed over me. The knots in my stomach slipped free. I was all in, 100 percent.

Wildly eager to see and touch my beautiful girls again, to hear their voices and laughter, I squeezed Mike's hand as we descended over the long glittering arms of the Dnieper River into Kyiv. After driving three hundred miles from their home in Belarus, Zoya, Ivan, Vika, and Maria would be there to greet us.

I tried to imagine how the girls had changed. They were now almost nineteen years old, studying at a college in Minsk, sharing a small apartment in the city with some of their classmates, and working as interns in a bank. The monthly stipend they received was small—the equivalent of fifty US dollars—but, in a country with constant inflation, it helped their family to make ends meet. Would I recognize them? Would the bond between us still feel strong after a separation of six years? Due to their busy schedules and ours, communication between us had been sparse since their last visit.

When the captain announced we were cleared for landing, I turned to Alex and Ella, seated across the aisle.

"We're really here!" I gasped.

My thoughts drifted to Zoya as we touched down. Though this would be our first introduction to her and Ivan in person, I felt as if I already knew them from the letters she and I had exchanged for ten years. Now, it would be impossible for us to converse without one of the girls translating every word. Would the language barrier create a painfully awkward gap between Zoya and me? I didn't want that to minimize or distort the close bond that had grown between us from a distance.

The long line through passport control moved glacially slow. When my passport finally was stamped, I charged to the baggage claim area, planning to snatch up our luggage and speed my way through customs. But there was a glitch. One of our bags was missing—the one containing the gifts we'd brought for the Petrovy family.

"It can't be lost!" I insisted.

I flashed on the black duffel the girls had always carried to Seattle filled with gifts for us. The thought of showing up on their side of the bridge empty-handed threw me into a tizzy. Gift giving was an important part of this family's culture, but my distress involved more than that. Unconsciously, I had hoped those gifts would offset whatever etiquette faux pas I blundered into. In a culture I didn't understand, so much remained beyond my control. Gift giving was one thing I had been certain I could manage. Now even that had slipped outside my control.

"They'll find it eventually," Mike reassured me with the confidence of a seasoned US business traveler. Scanning the room for the Ukrainian Airline office, he appeared utterly confused by signs he couldn't decipher. This was our first trip to Eastern Europe. His years of traveling were of no help to him in this part of the world. Though we'd spent hours studying the Cyrillic alphabet in preparation for the trip, he needed help to find the office and report a missing bag.

When Mike explained our situation to Alex, Alex blinked his eyes and shook his head. "Miii-chael, bag is gone," he said, dragging out the first syllable for emphasis. I heard pity in his voice. I didn't know if he felt sorry we'd lost the gifts or sorry that Mike couldn't accept the loss and go on. As though helping Mike to see the bitter truth, he added, "Don't bother making report. They will not find your bag."

"They'll find it!" Mike insisted. Expecting the same sort of service he was accustomed to at home, he added, "I'm not leaving here until I talk to someone who can get the wheels turning." He was so adamant that Alex finally humored him.

"Okay. I go with you, explain for you situation."

The clerk who took the report promised to contact Mike when the bag was located. Once again, Alex wanted to prevent Mike from grasping false hope. "This is Ukraine, not United States. You will never see bag again," he warned Mike after they left the office.

One bag short, we headed off to reunite with our Belarusian family. A rush of adrenaline shot through me as we stepped through automatic sliding doors into the chaos of people awaiting arrivals. I spotted Vika beaming at me from across the room. Standing next to her, on tiptoes, Maria waved with both hands, arms raised above the crowd. I walked toward them as though moving in a dream. The sea of people between me and the girls seemed to part by some invisible force. When we were almost close enough to touch, a scream of joy erupted out of me. Maria grabbed me and smashed her lips into mine. Struggling to keep my balance, I flashed back to a memory of eight-year-old Maria sliding across the wood floor of my living room in her stockinged feet and slamming into me with a smooch.

When Maria released me, Vika quietly stepped in and handed me a bouquet of deep red long-stemmed roses, a traditional Belarusian welcome gift. Her sapphire eyes gleamed.

"For you, Gail."

Wearing black eyeliner and her hair now dyed dark brown, she resembled Cleopatra more than the zealous little girl I remembered prancing around in my shoes with a mink pelt wrapped around her neck. Now, wearing lime-green wedge-heeled sandals, and with her dark hair spilling over her shoulders, Vika still was yin to Maria's yang. Immersed in the scent of roses, we savored a sweet embrace.

Next, I turned my attention to the short woman with a warm, youthful glow standing beside Vika. I recognized Zoya from the photos I'd seen. Embracing me with her chestnut eyes, she reached for me.

"Gail!" she cried.

I stepped into Zoya's arms and hugged her like a long-lost sister. After our long and comfortable embrace, Maria introduced me to her father.

"Gail, this Papa."

My Cold War impressions of Soviet men collided with reality when he wrapped me in a salt-of-the-earth hug. He was not a stoic man, as I'd expected. Tears of happiness clung to the corners of his gray-green eyes. Soon I would learn that he, like Alex and all of the Ukrainian and Belarusian men I would soon meet, was strong and gentle, proud of his ability to survive every storm, and filled with warmth.

I had heard that excessive radiation exposure had prematurely aged the liquidators who had been responsible for the cleanup of the Chernobyl explosion. But forty-seven-year-old Ivan, dressed in a short-sleeved buttoned shirt and black pants, appeared youthful and fit, like an ordinary man in the prime of his life. Yet, I knew his life had been anything but ordinary.

Our flock huddled together talking in two languages at once until Alex raised his voice above the din to capture our attention.

"Davay!" Come on. A bulging duffel bag hung from each of his shoulders. "Car is waiting outside. Driver leave if we not come." He had arranged for an extra car to transfer some of us and our luggage to our rental apartment in the city.

When we stepped outside to blue sky and sunshine, Vika laced her fingers through mine and ushered me to her father's car. As my hand melted into hers, all my concerns about feeling close disappeared like a pinch of salt in a cup of broth. Ivan and Mike lifted our bags into the trunk of Ivan's compact car while Alex, Ella, and Maria settled into the hired car.

As we whizzed along a busy, tree-lined boulevard, I expected to see a world completely foreign to me. Instead, the area reminded me of the outskirts of Seattle but without the hills. It was modern and orderly until we got close to the heart of the city, where the confusion and congestion reminded me of New York City. Ivan maneuvered through the knots of traffic and stopped in front of an old red-brick apartment building at 17 Basseinaya Street. Blocking traffic, he double-parked. Frustrated drivers blasted their horns as we jumped out of the car and unloaded our baggage.

"This way," said Alex. Ella and Maria stood next to him, waiting for us.

We followed Alex through an archway to the back of the building to meet the rental agent. After he and Alex exchanged greetings, the young man led us through an open doorway into total darkness. Trying to follow, I stumbled over bricks crumbling on the floor. *What in the world have we gotten ourselves into?* I wondered. As we turned a corner, a sliver of light showed through a window, exposing an elevator—a rickety-looking cage of metal bars. The contraption triggered my fear of elevators, which ordinarily troubled me only when I was closed inside alone.

"We go to floor seven," Alex explained. "Top floor—the best!"

"Who wants to take the stairs with me?" I asked, hoping I wouldn't have to choose between climbing the stairs alone or risking my life in a cage.

"Let's put all the bags in the elevator with Alex," Mike suggested. "The rest of us can take the stairs and help unload." I breathed a sigh of relief.

Halfway up the dimly lit concrete stairwell, we trooped by a man asleep on a landing. A whiff of urine gagged me as we turned the corner and kept climbing. *No different than many places in downtown Seattle*, I reminded myself. By the time we reached the seventh floor, I was prepared for the worst—but we stepped into a modern two-bedroom apartment with Asian decor, an open kitchen, a large jetted tub, and two balconies.

On the small balcony off the kitchen, a picturesque view of ordinary life in Kyiv greeted me. Strung from the back windows of old multi-storied apartment buildings, lines of laundry blew in the hot breeze like strings of prayer flags. A greenbelt of trees softened the city's sounds. In the distance, a cluster of skyscrapers seemed to inhabit a different world.

After a moment of quiet solitude, I joined Ella on the balcony overlooking Basseinaya, where the traffic noise was loud and constant. Cranes towered over buildings under construction in every direction. To me, they were signs of a growing economy.

Across the street, a huge billboard dominated by a helicopter and a rugged Marlboro-type man caught my eye. The caption was written in Cyrillic.

"What does that sign say?" I asked Ella.

Staring at the sign, Ella paused. A shadow crossed her face. "This say, 'Real man buy helicopter.'"

"Really?" I was incredulous. Wasn't Ukraine a poor country struggling to get its feet on the ground? I couldn't imagine any country where that billboard would make sense.

"This what is now. Rich people buy helicopter," said Ella. I didn't yet understand the sadness in her voice.

"Before Soviet Union collapse," Ella continued, "everybody poor but more stable. After Soviet Union break up, the factory where I worked closed because Russia stopped supplying materials. Then no jobs. This is why we left."

Where Mike and I saw signs of capitalism—as we knew it—trying to flourish in a new democracy, Ella saw instability and signs of an oligarchy-driven form of capitalism. Her loved ones in Ukraine had all but given up any hope that the political and economic revitalization of Ukraine would improve their difficult lives and give rise to a middle class.

"So many changes," Ella sighed. I couldn't have imagined that ten years later I would see an oligarchy come into view in my own country.

When Ella and I stepped back inside, Alex threw up his hands. "One toilet! I ask for two!" he lamented.

I knew that one toilet wasn't a problem for him or Ella. Before moving to the United States they had no indoor plumbing. His disappointment stemmed from feeling responsible for Mike's and my comfort and meeting what he assumed were our American standards. He frowned apologetically.

"Maybe you not comfortable," he said, as though he'd let us down.

"One bathroom is plenty," I reassured him. "We grew up in one-bathroom homes, and our parents grew up with outhouses." I dismissed his worry with a wave of my hand. On this trip, I would have used a bucket, if necessary.

When Ivan returned from parking the car, we all sat in the living room while he and Zoya discussed our itinerary with Ella and Alex. I tried to track the conversation, but it bounced between them so rapidly that I couldn't understand a word. I assumed they were talking about meeting our train in Belarus and how long we would stay. Overcome by jet lag, I closed my eyes and rested until Alex made an announcement.

"New plan!" It was the first of many times he would announce a *new plan* during our travels together. "After Kyiv, we will all stay with Babushka in her village one hour from here. Ella and I will stay one night then go to my sister in Vinnytsia. Mike and Gail, you stay two nights with Babushka, then Maria and Vika will take the train with you to Belarus. After Belarus, they go back to work and you take train to Vinnytsia. I will get you hotel."

I was thrilled to receive the unexpected invitation to meet Babushka and stay in her home, but the rest of the plan came as a shock. *Maria and Vika will escort us to Belarus instead of Ella? Our lives will be in the hands of teenagers wearing minuscule skirts and off-the-shoulder tops with their cleavage and pierced belly buttons exposed!*

"Gail, it's okay I not go to Belarus with you? You be okay?" Ella asked.

I paused, thinking about taking the train back to Kyiv and on to Vinnytsia, without the girls, when we left Belarus. Then, I heard the voice of the guidebook author whispering in my ear. *As long as you're not on a blacklist of political activists, you'll be fine.*

"I'll be fine!" I answered, feeling thankful that, since living in Minsk, the girls had acquired cell phones. After my initial shock wore off, that affirmation began to ring true. It *was* okay. *At least they can call for backup if anything goes sideways.*

The twins and their parents left to stay with Babushka, giving us time to recover from our trip. Maria left her cell phone with Mike so he could be reached if our bag was located. Reeling from sleep deprivation and a blur of time zone changes, we crawled into bed early. When the phone rang, about midnight, it startled us awake. Mike answered and listened to a man speaking Russian. Then he jumped out of bed and grabbed his pants and shirt.

"Where are you going?"

"Downstairs. I think some guy from the airport is here with our bag."

"You're not sure?"

"Nope. It could have been one of Maria's friends calling. But I'm pretty sure he said McCormick, and *samolet*." *Airplane*. He headed down the stairs.

Awakened by the commotion, Alex popped out of his bedroom to see what was going on.

"Someone called. Mike went downstairs to see if our suitcase has been delivered," I explained.

Alex's face twisted in alarm. "I better go, just in case," he said, rushing out the door. Moments later, they returned with the missing bag.

"Only because you are American," said Alex as he went back to bed.

Happily tucked into that city of three million people, with horns blowing, trucks roaring, and traffic growling all night, I drifted back into a deep and dreamy sleep.

CHAPTER 21

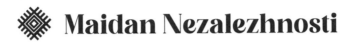 # Maidan Nezalezhnosti

Ukraine

With just one day to introduce Mike and me to the city of Kyiv, Alex and Ella rose at 5:00 a.m. While we still slept, they quietly slipped out of the apartment and roamed the streets to grasp the lay of the land. Ella had been to the capital city only once before, at sixteen years old, on a trip with her father to visit relatives. Neither she nor Alex had had the opportunity nor financial resources to explore their own country while living there. Now, as they visited their motherland for the first time since they had emigrated to the United States, sleep took a back seat to feasting on a culture that was both familiar and new to them.

I awakened to a Ukrainian blue sky above and a traffic frenzy below. Rattling around the kitchen, Mike was searching for a coffeemaker.

"Where are Ella and Alex?"

"Don't know," answered Mike. "Making a coffee run, maybe."

Soon, Vika and Maria's cousin Vasyl dropped the twins off, as planned, to spend the day with us in Kyiv; the three of them had spent the night in the village where his parents and their *babushka* lived. The tanned, long-legged twins made their entrance wearing their nano skirts and sunglasses. Then Alex and Ella returned carrying a bag of groceries and a cardboard tray of steaming paper cups, their faces glowing with pride and excitement.

"I smell coffee!" Mike sang out.

"Of course!" Ella smiled and unpacked the coffee, bread, cheese, and pastries they'd brought back for breakfast.

"We have plan!" Alex informed us. "We hire guide to make for us tour of city. Is very good. Special bus just for us," he enthused. "Everybody sit beside window." He ended with a sweep of his upheld palms in the air, like the conductor of an orchestra.

"Sounds great! What time?" Mike asked.

"In afternoon," said Ella. "First I go with you and Gail to train station to see about your tickets to Belarus. Vasyl drive us there."

Still recovering from jet lag, we enjoyed a leisurely breakfast. The coffee drinkers savored their caffeine. Then we took our time preparing for a day of sightseeing. Thinking we were waiting for Vasyl to pick us up, I kept expecting his knock at the door.

"What time is Vasyl coming?" I finally asked, assuming he'd gone home to his apartment and was coming back for us.

"He waiting downstairs in the car," answered Vika, sitting with her legs crossed, admiring her freshly painted fingernails.

"He's been waiting for us since you and Maria arrived?" I asked, astonished. "I'm so sorry we've kept him waiting this long!"

"Is okay, Gail. No problem," she assured me.

In my life, being made to wait unnecessarily could be a source of conflict. If Mike and I agreed to meet at a specific time and he was more than ten minutes late, I felt both disrespected and scared. One minute, I'd imagine him struck by a bus, bleeding to death. The next minute, I wanted to lash out at him for losing track of the time.

After several of Maria and Vika's other family members had also waited long periods for us—without our knowing it—I wondered if I was witnessing a different approach to life, one not driven by the clock. I admired that kind of patience and sense of duty, in contrast to the constant rushing in my consumer-driven culture. I wanted to believe Ukrainians chose to master the art of waiting as a noble cause. But I'd never experienced the kinds of hardships that had shaped their behavior. The legacy they carried from centuries of famines, invasions, and unpredictability had a powerful impact I could hardly imagine. Ella and Alex had shared memories with me of waiting in lines for hours to purchase small rations of food during the Soviet era. For them, waiting had not been optional, nor was it a cause. It was life.

Vasyl drove us to the station and waited another long stretch of time while we finished our business. Then he dropped us off on Khreschatyk Boulevard, Kyiv's busy main thoroughfare in the heart of the city, to meet Alex and the twins at Maidan Nezalezhnosti—Independence Square.

"This is where Orange Revolution happen," said Ella as we popped out of the car.

The street ran through the middle of the expansive square, a hardscape of wide brick walkways, cascading staircases, triumphal arches, fountains, and monuments. Green trees on the perimeter and small flower gardens added color to the neutral canvas, like bold-colored stitches on a *rushnyk*, the traditional Ukrainian ritual cloth.

"Wasn't that in 2005? When Yanukovych stole the presidential election from Viktor Yushchenko?" Mike asked.

"Yes," confirmed Ella. "Election rigged. So much corruption. Because of Orange Revolution, they make new, fair election, and Yushchenko won."

Just then we heard Maria's voice. "Ella! Gail!" She and Vika were standing in a shallow stream of water flowing gently down a staircase in the square, their sandals dangling from their hands.

As I smiled and waved, I thought about them as little girls calling me into the water at Lake Washington on their first trip to Seattle, ten years earlier. Then I focused on them now—Vika wearing a fitted red blouse with a plunging neckline, and Maria's belly button peeking out below her off-the-shoulder blouse. Juggling the past with the present in a compressed timeline of images, I hardly noticed the backdrop of Stalinist architecture surrounding us.

"Take shoes off!" called Maria.

I wanted to fling my sandals off and join the girls but wasn't sure that would be appropriate behavior for a grown woman—a foreign tourist—in downtown Kyiv. I remembered seeing this iconic place on the news, jammed with pro-democracy protesters wearing orange bands, refusing to give up, their sleeping tents sagging in deep drifts of snow. *Out of respect, should I keep my shoes on my feet?* I remembered when once, on a train in Switzerland, I had put my feet up to rest on an empty seat facing me; a chagrined Swiss woman, seated across the aisle, politely handed me a newspaper to place under my shoes to keep the upholstery clean. I would try to never make that mistake again, to be a careless guest in a foreign culture.

"Water very nice," Vika encouraged me.

I glanced at Ella. Eager to share Ukraine's hard-won independence with her American friend, she gave me a quick nod. "Let's go!" We slipped off our sandals and joined the girls in something akin to a baptism, a rite of freedom so apt, so fresh.

"Would you have done this before Ukraine's independence?" I asked Ella.

"No. Not allowed," she said. Those kinds of restrictions still governed Vika and Maria's lives in Belarus. They were straddling two worlds and understood the rules of both.

As the cool water washed over our feet, Vika clasped my hand, and I reached out my other hand to connect with Maria. A current flowed effortlessly between us and filled me with a familiar sense of oneness, the same feeling I had experienced with the girls when they were kids visiting America. Now, on their end of the bridge we'd built, I was giddy, caught up in the zeal of early independence—of Ukraine and my twins who had reached the threshold of adulthood.

That day, I took for granted the freedom we celebrated in the Maidan. Had I known that fifteen years later Russia would pound Kyiv with bombs and missiles, I would have kissed the ground and wept.

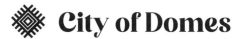 City of Domes

Ukraine

"My name is Boris." *Rhymes with police*, I noted silently, to help me remember how to correctly pronounce our handsome young guide's name. Standing in the front of the minibus, facing us, his tall, lean frame nearly touched the ceiling. Studying his warm face with its five-o-clock shadow, I guessed he was thirtyish. It wouldn't take long to realize he was a visionary with a passion for Kyiv and for democracy. His introduction to the city began there, at Independence Square, with his own heartfelt experience of the Orange Revolution.

"Never before had I experienced such a strong sense of community and peace, everyone helping to care for each other in the cold, sharing their food, their fires, whatever they had." He spoke from his heart rather than a script.

"During the revolution," Boris continued, "anywhere from half a million to one million citizens protested each day. It was one of the biggest peaceful protests that had ever taken place in the world, and one of the most successful." He exuded gratitude and humility.

When Boris spoke, I heard the voice of a confident leader. The voice of a new generation of changemakers with the audacity to believe in non-violence, truth, cooperation, and equality over dominance. A sudden burst of emotion gathered in my throat and urged me to cry. It was hope rising, but I held those tears back. *Yes! The world is desperate for people in power who embody wisdom, justice, and compassion.*

Outside my window, I scanned the square, Kyiv's center stage for displays of political might as well as unrest. People strolled by with the ease of those who feel free and safe. Is that what Ella and Alex and the twins saw too? Or did they see people caught in a tumultuous transition from communism to a society where *anything* goes? Years later, I would think about Boris. *Has he lost hope? Is he alive?*

When we left the Maidan, Boris showed us a city of domes, the signature of holy places kissing the sky in Kyiv.

Though the Byzantine and Baroque cathedrals impressed me with their masterful artwork, size, and antiquity, it was the domes that captured my affection. In rich hues of blue, green, and brilliant gold, those mystical orbs spoke to me of the feminine, earth-based practices that preceded patriarchal religions. My favorite was the onion dome, with its deep sensual curves.

Kyiv's cathedrals were the treasure troves of her long history. Inside their walls, centuries of prayers and sorrows hung in the air. I wanted to feel the touch of God as I stood in the sanctuaries. Instead, I found myself feeling disconnected from Spirit and overwhelmed by the profusion of elaborate icons and gilding. I couldn't make sense of the unease I felt until Boris explained that the ambiance was designed, at least in part, to intimidate potential invaders with a show of wealth and power. Then I understood, it was that imbalance— extolling the dominance of the masculine—that stood between Mystery and me. The feminine side of God—grace, humility, equality, compassion—was overshadowed, profoundly out of balance. I needed that balance to feel whole. Holy.

I understood we had signed up for a historical tour, not a transcendent experience. But I wanted more than history. I wanted to see Vika and Maria light up the way they had when we sang chants and lit prayer candles at the Taizé service we attended together in Seattle. I wanted to know how my Jewish friend Ella felt as we toured these Christian cathedrals. Was she remembering her ancestors who were killed during the pogroms in Ukraine?

As I followed in the footsteps of Ukraine's spiritual ancestors with a heavy heart, I suddenly encountered the Blessed Mother standing in front of me on a pedestal, gazing at me with compassion. As I paused in her gentle stillness, a spaciousness opened in my chest. It was the same feeling that comes to me when I gaze into a night sky and see the Milky Way. Now, I took a deep breath, basking in the mystical connection I felt to Mary. For me, she was starlight illuminating the dark—always present but not always seen and felt. The weight on my heart began to lift as though she had wrapped me in a shawl of peace. I felt grateful for Mary's presence, bridging the gap between ancient matriarchal spirituality and the patriarchal religions practiced today. In my eyes, she was the feminine face of God.

After our immersion in cathedrals, Boris took us to see another artifact of Ukraine's ancient history—four pagan statues standing outside a historical museum. Though I knew that Ukraine and Belarus still honored ties with their pagan history, the presence of these deities in a predominantly Orthodox city surprised me. I hurried off the bus and approached two totems that towered over me with droopy breasts and wide hips, their palms resting low on their bellies the way women do when carrying a child in their womb.

I began to realize that the feminine counterbalance to

the dominance of the masculine in Kyiv was hidden everywhere in plain sight. In cathedrals and relics. Even in the
soul of a tour guide and revolutionary.

At the end of our excursion, we dragged our weary
selves back to our apartment for a nap before dinner.

"Who will wake us up?" asked Ella.

"The goddesses." I smiled.

After a short rest, I knew I needed soothing water to rejuve-
nate me. So I ran hot water into the tub to soak my aching
feet. Sitting on the edge of the tub, leaning against the wall
behind me, I closed my eyes. Images and colors of Kyiv tumbled through my mind like bits of dreams. Brilliant flashes
of gold domes and crosses. Crumbling red brick pavers and
doorways. Skyscrapers under construction. Chaotic traffic.
Trees. Gardens. Sprinkles of blue, yellow, white, and green
cathedrals.

My daydream ended abruptly when Maria startled me.
"You soak feet, Gail?"

"Yes. Come and join me!" Vika arrived right behind her.

It was a rare and welcome opportunity for me to spend
time alone with the twins. There was no other place where I
would have been happier than I was in that moment, sitting
with my girls on the edge of the pie-shaped jacuzzi tub with
our feet immersed, once again, in healing water.

"Ohhh. This feel very good," moaned Maria. "Maybe
I not go to dinner. No more walking."

"What about you, Vika?" I asked. "Your feet must hurt
from walking all day in those wedge-heeled sandals."

"No. My feet very good," claimed Vika, flipping her long
hair over her shoulder.

Maria began singing in a soft voice, then launched
into a pop star performance with exaggerated eye and lip

movements, her head rocking from left to right in sync with her arms, waving above her head. Enjoying her silly mood, Vika and I giggled. Going for a bigger reaction, Maria built up steam and pulled a retractable showerhead out of the wall and held it in front of her, like a microphone on a long cord. Still keeping her voice low, she shook her long golden hair into a frenzy, pretending to belt her song into the tub apparatus until all three of us were bent in half, trying to muffle our laughing.

When we caught our breath, Maria's mood quickly turned solemn, reminding me of her as a little girl, when her moods could shift abruptly. She leaned toward her sister. Now, she and Vika joined their voices in a passionate duet. This time, they didn't hold back.

Rising and falling, the girls' soulful voices carried through the walls and doorways. Alex, Ella, and Mike stirred from their slumber, awakened by the song of the goddesses.

CHAPTER 23

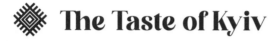 **The Taste of Kyiv**

Ukraine

Our night out on the town in Kyiv began with dinner at a brightly lit, cafeteria-style restaurant just beginning to make a name for itself, Puzata Khata. "Means *full belly*," said Ella. Known for its "homestyle classic Ukrainian cuisine" and "democratic" prices, according to reviews, Ella and Alex had decided it was a perfect place for us to eat that wouldn't blow their budget.

This was a first for all of us.

When Alex and Ella had lived in Ukraine, restaurants were for the elite. They had never seen the inside of a restaurant before they emigrated. When Mike and I first met them, four years after their move to Seattle, they still had never indulged, even though eating out was common in the United States. With the money they saved by Ella making all their meals, they were able to achieve their American dream of purchasing their own home.

Mike and I often frequented cafés and restaurants in Seattle and on our travels, and we had taken Vika and Maria out to eat during their visits to the United States. The first restaurant we dined in together was in Seattle's International

District, where we'd gone to a Chinese parade, part of
Seattle's summer Seafair festival. Unaccustomed to Asian
food, the twins ate little more than white rice with ketchup
smeared on it—with chopsticks. Now, at Puzata Khata, we
were about to share with them their first restaurant meal in
Eastern Europe.

With Alex in the lead, we streamed into Puzata Khata
on Basseinaya Street. A savory blend of garlic, bread, and
chicken perfumed the air as we picked up trays and formed
a line. Stretched out before us, behind a clear partition, was
a long countertop covered with serving trays and chafing
dishes laden with food.

"You can see *every*thing," Alex beamed. "Make it easy
for you." He was a man who would turn water into wine
for you, if he could.

"Help steer me away from anything that includes jellied
meat, pickled fish, or caviar," I whispered to Mike, eyeball-
ing the huge spread. Upon closer inspection, I realized most
of the choices were familiar and appealing.

"*Golubtsi, pozhaluysta*," I said awkwardly to the
matronly woman who stood behind the counter waiting to
dish my food. *Cabbage rolls, please.* "*Yi kottlet*," I added,
pointing to a pan of steaming chicken breasts, pounded thin
and fried. Unable to decipher a word I'd spoken, she looked
at me askance. Chuckling, Vika stepped in to translate.

Gathered around a table for six, we ate potluck style,
passing dishes back and forth to share. Cheesy crepes. Cabbage salad. Potato pancakes with sour cream. Rolled pork
stuffed with herbs. A dreamy slice of cake made with hazel-
nuts, cocoa, meringue, and buttercream.

After the strain of communicating all day with a mix
of languages and translations that didn't always hit the
mark, we kept our dinner conversation simple, reverting to
sentences of three words or less, requiring no translation.

Vkusno. Tasty. You try *ryba*? Fish? No, thank you. Mmm. Sauce very good! Sour cream, *pozhaluysta.*

Hot, fresh, and laced with dill, the flavors brought back to me the cozy contentment I associated with eating at Ella's table. Even she and Alex gave the food at Puzata Khata their stamp of approval.

There was a handful of other people seated in the restaurant, mostly young people wearing suits or casual office attire. Later, Ella confirmed they were most likely locals, young professionals working in the city. Casual restaurants couldn't rely on travelers, she said, because Ukraine wasn't yet known as a tourist destination. Puzata Khata was a testament to the growth of a new class of workers taking shape along with a free enterprise system.

But Puzata Khata's true personality was revealed in the women's restroom, where the twins, Ella, and I were greeted by walls of brilliant red tiles.

"Look!" said Vika, pointing our attention to a whimsical sketch hung in a frame on the glossy tiles next to the sink. It was the backside of a nude woman shaped like a chunky onion dome.

"A one-picture art gallery!" I said as we all laughed.

"I could live in this room!" remarked Maria. It was the size of a small studio apartment, bigger and brighter than her current room in Minsk. With flush toilets and a good supply of toilet paper, it was a ten on a 0–10 scale of public rest stops we would encounter on this trip.

From Puzata Khata we walked to a subway stop, descended on a long escalator, and zipped downtown to join the late-night promenade of Kyivans on Khreschatyk Boulevard. A warm breeze made it perfect for sauntering among sultry women on the arms of adoring men, families enjoying a reprieve from stuffy apartments, and young people out to see and be seen by each other.

Ella and Alex stepped into the parade with the ease of belonging. Engaged in the familiar rhythm of people who understood their history and shared their language and culture, their faces seemed to glow from the inside. Restored by the power of ritual, they were no longer tourists in their native land. They had truly come home. There was no doubt in my mind, I was witnessing them becoming one with their tribe.

At first, I was an outsider, satisfied with my role as an observer. Then I sensed a shift. I could taste Kyiv, a mixture of vibrant and earthy, newborn and ancient, champagne and vodka, high heels and sneakers. Suddenly, I was a participant in something greater than me. For a mysterious moment, my heart opened, and I felt connected to humanity. Feeling grateful, I locked arms with Ella.

"In Ukraine, everyone walk at night," she said. "Not like Seattle. When we move there we feel so alone. Everyone drive cars. Children stay inside. Alex want to know, 'Where all the people?'" For Ella, the stroll was a loving embrace, a welcome home.

The twins carried themselves with the confidence of queens. Heads high. Shoulders back. Long strides. Vika's nose tipped slightly skyward. Maria's blouse pulled way off her shoulder. Their maturity both shocked me and filled me with pride. I hoped that their trips to Seattle, learning to navigate in a foreign land at an early age, had contributed to their sense of comfort in the world. And I hoped it had been internalized so deeply that they would always find their way through any storms they encountered in life.

After we had walked for more than an hour, the air cooled. My transcendent moment passed. And I was reeling from a sensory overload. Twilight's magic gave way to the glare of billboards looming overhead, plastered with diamonds and thousand-dollar handbags. Big black SUVs with tinted windows and other lavish cars streaked by in a steady stream. Even Maria and Vika were tired and ready to leave.

Traveling back to our apartment where cozy beds awaited us, the subway nearly rocked me to sleep with Vika's head resting on my shoulder. I never dreamed that would be my last visit to Kyiv, or that the subway would one day double as a bomb shelter, protecting the city's residents from missiles.

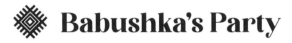 Babushka's Party

Ukraine

White storks nest in trees in Vasilki, a Ukrainian village of one-story houses, dirt roads, and a tiny market where residents purchase bread, cheese, ice cream bars, cigarettes, and headscarves. One of many villages built in the 1980s by the Soviets to house Chernobyl families, it felt like a place time had forgotten when we arrived in 2007.

I recognized Babushka's home from the photograph the twins had shown me ten years earlier, on their first trip to Seattle. In front of the house were the same weathered fence and old wooden bench where Babushka and her family had posed for that picture. Seeing in real life the little house with its tin roof, sky-blue window frames, white diamond motifs, and a peacock-blue gable, I felt as though I had stepped into a fairy tale.

We arrived with Ella, Alex, and the twins in two cars, one driven by Ivan, the second one by his brother-in-law. The moment we pulled up in front of the house, a hearty woman wearing a gray skirt, printed blouse, and a gold flowered headscarf tied under her chin marched through the gate to greet us. I recognized Babushka's face and shape from her photo, but her straight back, brisk stride, and regal air caught me by surprise. She was not the defeated, hunched widow I had expected. Without a word, she grabbed Mike and me into her arms and held us tight against her ample breasts.

"*Ya* Galyna," she said when she finally released us. *I'm Galyna.*

Strong and sturdy from planting potatoes and heaving pig slop, sixty-seven-year-old Babushka had a lot to teach me about the character and hardiness of Ukrainian women. Her solid voice and vigorous embrace told me she was strong in body, mind, and spirit. Looking into her deep gray-green eyes, I felt a kinship with her.

As Babushka turned and led us toward the gate, a rooster crowed and a goose squawked as if they, too, recognized the significance of the bond deepening between our two families. A parade of cows moseyed by on their way to pasture. Tottering along behind them, an old woman waved a stick to keep the animals from straying.

Inside the gate, a carpet of wild strawberries covered the ground. Cherries hung on trees like hundreds of kisses dangling from branches. Zoya, along with Ivan's sister and a couple of neighbors, stood waiting to meet us. A hush fell over them as we approached. I wondered if we were the first Americans some of them had ever met face-to-face.

Zoya stood at the head of the line. "Hello!" she called, breaking the ice.

"*Zdravstvuyte!*" I replied. *Hello.*

A nervous elation ran through me as the procession of hugs and handshakes pulled us toward the concrete stoop with two steps leading to the front door of the house. With the twins at our heels, we followed their grandmother up the stairs to a doorway draped with white lace panels. Thrilled to wed us to their family, the girls glowed like bridesmaids when we reached the threshold. Babushka smiled and led us into the cool, dark entry of her home. Fragrances of earth, broth, and bread mingled in the air.

With an elegant sweep of her hand, Vika directed our attention to a cozy bedroom on our right. "This you, Gail and Mike." She beamed as if she were showing us to a honeymoon suite.

It was a room with twin beds where Babushka watched television, cross-stitched, and slept. Her bold floral and geometric designs covered the pillows on the beds. Stoic ancestors peered down at us from pictures hung on the walls with cross-stitched runners draped over their white wood frames like shawls. Pink, red, yellow, green, blue, and black stitches sprinkled the room like confetti.

"*Krasivaya!*" I remarked. *Beautiful.* From the girls' giggles, I surmised that my pronunciation was incorrect, but I was determined to use what little Russian I could.

Taking the lead again, Galyna showed us to an adjoining room where a clay igloo-shaped structure, connected to a wall by a flat, enclosed bridge, occupied most of the space. She touched the clay with her hand and nodded, signaling us to follow suit. Curious, I touched the dome.

"Yikes!" I yelped, yanking my hand away before my skin burned. "It's hot!"

"*Da!*" Galyna's eyes twinkled. Motioning for us to follow, she walked back out into the hall. There, through an opening in the wall, we saw food cooking on a bed of red-hot coals inside the dome. I inhaled a deep breath of a tantalizing aroma.

"Papa and Uncle make this oven for Babushka," said Maria, a replica, she explained, of the oven Babushka had to leave behind when she was evacuated from her beloved home on a riverbank near Chernobyl. Babushka listened intently as Maria spoke. Though she couldn't understand

English, she sensed Maria had forgotten to mention an important detail. Before we moved on, she spoke to Maria.

"She want me say this number one oven in Vasilki," relayed Maria.

"It's the best oven in Vasilki?"

"*Da*," confirmed Maria.

"*Da*," repeated Babushka, her face lit with pleasure.

Fully present to the wonder of the moment, I stood in the heart of the former USSR basking in the warmth of an old-world Soviet woman and her clay oven. Gazing at the three women beside me, I felt as though I'd entered a delightful time warp. Babushka, with hair poking out from under her scarf, looked like she could have just stepped out of the nineteenth century. Beside her stood Maria wearing a halter top, faded denim shorts not more than six inches long, and a silver ring protruding from her navel. Vika wore shorts almost identical to Maria's and a T-shirt that said, written in English, AHEAD OF HER TIME. I was a US baby boomer with a Baggallini travel bag slung over my shoulder. The past and the future swirled together like a post-modern family portrait.

Satisfied that I understood the oven's stature, Babushka led us past her tiny kitchen—where I caught a glimpse of a pot simmering over a flame on the stove—to the back room of the house. The girls' cousins, Vasyl and his younger brother Denys, were in the room, threading an extension cord through the window to hang a light bulb in a tree. The boys made eye contact with us and flashed warm smiles. The air rippled with excitement in anticipation of the party Babushka had planned for that night in honor of her American guests.

"*Privet!*" said both young men. *Hi.*

"*Privet!*" I answered.

Through the windowpane, I saw Ivan and two helpers outside. The men were digging a fire pit and assembling makeshift benches out of planks of wood held up by chairs on each end of a table standing under the tree. On the periphery stood a fenced area in front of a small sagging barn; inside the pen, a light-skinned pig was rooting around. On the opposite side of the yard, dill and vegetables grew in a garden. Staged against the backdrop of a potato field with dark furrowed rows and green plants already knee-high, the setting made me feel like I had time-traveled back to my grandparents' farm.

In the room where we were standing, a Turkish-style rug in shades of brown hung on one wall, reminiscent of the ancient Silk Road trade routes still connecting Eastern Europe with Asia. I'd never seen a rug used as insulation and wall art, but I would see this feature in every home I visited in Ukraine and Belarus.

The furnishings included a sofa, a wood table and stools, a buffet, and a wardrobe. The buffet and wardrobe appeared to provide the only storage space in the house. There were no closets, and no bathroom. I couldn't imagine where Babushka kept all her shoes, clothes, coats, boots, linens, batteries, vases, and tchotchkes. Where were her suitcases, Christmas ornaments, and flashlights? A picture of the storage areas in my home flashed in my head, shelves and closets in every room, plus the garage and basement, all overflowing with more *stuff* than I could use. I cringed. Though I didn't consider myself overly materialistic, I had no idea how little I really needed.

After the house tour, Babushka joined Zoya in the kitchen to peel potatoes and chop garlic, dill, and cabbage from the garden while the twins took Mike and me outdoors to acquaint us with the loo. Situated over a pit dug behind the barn, it was a classic planked-wood one-seater outhouse stocked with squares of toilet paper. Air and light squeezed in through the cracks between the boards. I was relieved to discover there were no chemical deodorizers inside. There were no odors of any kind. Without leaving any trace of toxic chemicals that would make me ill, someone had cleaned that tiny latrine from top to bottom to make our visits to the throne more pleasant when nature called. For a person with environmental illness, this rated better than some four-star hotels.

After checking out the privy, we sauntered down the road—the equivalent of a long city block—to the well where every drop of water Babushka used to drink, clean, bathe, and cook had to be raised in a pail and carried home in pots.

"I show you," said Vika. She cranked the rope until the bucket appeared with water slopping over its rim. "You try? Is very good!" she assured us.

"I'll have some," Mike answered.

Vika poured water into his cupped hands then turned to me. "Gail?"

Normally I followed the recommendation that Americans drink only bottled water when visiting Eastern Europe, and most other countries, to avoid contaminants we're not accustomed to. But I made an exception because I didn't want to offend Vika, and the crystal-clear water, cold and fresh from the earth, looked mighty appealing in the heat.

"Sure!" I said, taking a leap of faith.

It wasn't the first health risk I'd taken on this trip, nor would it be the last. I'd already indulged in eating foods that included gluten and dairy products when temptation got the better of me. I also didn't want to disappoint Babushka or Zoya, who went to great effort and expense to prepare special dishes for us; I told myself that the amount of love that went into their work in the kitchen must have protective powers. I was traveling with supplements to support immunity and digestion, and I'd heard that some Americans found wheat and dairy products in Europe to be less allergenic (due to less processing and additives). Most importantly, I was certain the reactions I'd have wouldn't be life threatening. Fortunately, I made it through the trip without debilitating repercussions; the worst effects didn't hit until after I returned to Seattle.

"Water is *very* good," I agreed, slurping from my cupped hands. *How in the world does Babushka carry water home from the well when the ground is covered with snow and ice?* I wondered.

From the well, we walked around a bend where a deserted, one-story building with no windows came into view.

"Is *banya*," said Maria.

Ella had told me stories about going to the *banya* in her village when she lived in Ukraine. It was a public steam bath where, separated by gender, adults and children went to bathe, socialize, and improve their health. Every village worth its salt had a *banya*, she said.

This *banya* was "no good," explained Vika. The water pipes had broken years ago and never been repaired. I wondered how the people of Vasilki bathed in the winter. And, with no community hall, no church, and no banya, where did they gather?

We circled back and joined four generations of the Petrovy clan for an al fresco celebration as the sun dipped toward the horizon. Skewered pork sizzled over the fire pit as our party of sixteen adults and one baby sat shoulder to shoulder in the shade of the tree. Zoya ladled borscht into bowls and passed them around. Ivan pulled the hot skewers of meat from the coals and delivered them to our plates. Babushka suddenly cried, "Oy!" and rushed back into the house. When she returned, gripping a red polka-dotted teapot in one hand, the family howled with laughter.

Babushka ceremoniously lifted the teapot as though making a toast. "*Chai!*" she announced, causing another roar of laughter.

Confused, I turned to Maria.

"This Babushka vodka!" she explained, still laughing so hard I thought the silver ring protruding from her navel might pop out. "She make with potato."

With the aplomb and expertise of a master, Babushka started filling shot glasses with her home-brewed "*chai*" while Ivan passed the platter of homemade dill pickles—the vodka chasers.

Babushka picked up the shot glass in front of my plate and our eyes met. I held up my hand like a stop sign and smiled.

"*Niet, spacibo,*" I said. *No, thank you.*

Babushka nodded knowingly, as if she'd been fore-warned that I suffered with mysterious health issues that prevented me from drinking hard liquor. When it came to alcohol, I was a lightweight. I could sip a glass of wine with no regrets. After one shot of vodka, however, I'd soon be ready for bed, and I didn't want to miss a moment of this party. But I also didn't want to miss out on the homemade baby dill pickles, one of my favorite foods.

Banter filled the air as dishes of food made their way around the table. When the pickles reached me, I asked Ivan, "Can I eat pickles if I don't drink vodka?"

Ivan flashed a huge smile. His gold front tooth glittered. "You can eat *all* the pickles, if you want!" he answered in Russian.

Those sour pickles, reminiscent of the ones my aunt made when I was a child, did not disappoint. Neither did the borscht. When the beets, cabbage, and sour cream exploded in my mouth I wanted to scream, *This is the real thing! I'm eating borscht in Ukraine!*

I heaped my plate with cabbage salad laced with tangy moss-colored dill fresh from the garden, and homegrown potatoes boiled in a savory broth that invoked the com-fort, flavors, and scents of my grandmother's house in the 1950s. I cut into my pork, anticipating the delightful taste of its savory clear juice. When bright pink juice poured out instead, I stopped cutting and took a sharp breath.

The meat wasn't cooked enough for me to feel it was safe to eat, but I couldn't bring myself to ask Ivan to throw it back on the fire. Nor could I bring myself to waste the precious meat that had come from Babushka's labors, not from a grocery store. Every year she planted, hoed, and harvested two or more acres of potatoes to fatten a single pig in order to feed her family through the winter. After raising and butchering her porker, she canned the meat and stored it in an underground cellar. The pork on my plate could probably have fed her for at least a week. After considering the options, I said a silent prayer and ate the *shashlyk*, leaving just the rarest bits on my plate.

Conversation and vodka zipped around the table as the sun continued to drop. After a couple of shots of "*chai*," Babushka asked in her native tongue, "Can you find me a boyfriend in America?" Her green eyes danced with mischief.

Everyone guffawed as Vika translated my offer to place a personal ad in a Seattle newspaper. "Ukrainian *babushka* looking for love. Has pig. Will travel."

"*Yi chai!*" Babushka shot back, raising her teapot. *And tea!*

Imagining Babushka arriving at the airport in Seattle with a pig and a jar of her homemade vodka, we shared a good-hearted laugh. But I sensed that Babushka's humor concealed a part of her that missed her husband terribly, a part that was tired of lifting water from the well and carrying it alone, tired of hoeing potatoes and fattening pigs without her husband at her side. No one mentioned the cause of her husband's early death, only that he had worked as a bookkeeper at the Chernobyl power station and had stayed behind, after the evacuation, to help with the disposal of contaminated animals.

Completely at home in the spotlight, Galyna was made

for the role of matriarch. By personality, perseverance, and girth, Babushka was a giant living in a hobbit house.

When we finished eating, the sun had set, and the horizon was ablaze with color, a wide band of purple light with a narrow strip of coral stacked on top. As the luminous colors peaked and began to fade, Ivan hefted a green-and-black accordion onto his lap. Quiet fell among us as an ancient voice spilled through the bellows.

Babushka stood and began to sing a song filled with lament and sorrow. The creases in her face told a story of hardship and strength. Later I would learn that, as a child, she had survived the Nazi invasion of Ukraine during World War II by living in the forest.

Achingly beautiful, the music and Babushka's voice invoked the spirits of ancestors. Their lamentations poured out like healing water as every member of the family joined in singing. When the sea of pasture, fields, and forest grew darker, the arc of light from the bare bulb hung in the tree created an aura around our island of souls. I looked from face to face and saw the shine of unshed tears. A heaviness gathered around us.

I thought about the other villagers hearing this song. All of them had been evacuated from Chernobyl, ripped from the land their families had called home for generations. I thought about my own losses. My brother's death. Three pregnancy losses. The children and grandchildren I would never have. The toll chemicals had taken on my health.

Instead of sinking into grief, I felt the music lifting me in some mysterious way, as though I had listened for this song my whole life. It opened a door in me I hardly remembered was there. I pictured the Hawaiian guitar I had found years ago buried in my father's closet on the farm. How he had acquired it I never knew. To my knowledge, neither he nor my mother ever sang, or danced, or played music. Now, sitting at Babushka's table, I wished my father had brought that old guitar to life. I wished my family could have shared the unsung joys and sorrows in our hearts. Ecstasy, heartache, and awe slowly filled the awkward silence that had lived in me since childhood.

Then, without warning, Ivan launched into a lively tune that plucked us out of the past. Denys, a young man with a round face and rosy cheeks, locked arms with his father. Singing together, they pumped their arms and kicked their legs with gusto as the rest of us clapped and hollered. For me, a woman whose parents didn't even move their lips when the congregation sang in church, the change of ambiance was sudden and dramatic. The Petrovy family negotiated the rise and fall of emotion as if it were as natural to them as breathing. Their exuberance splashed in my heart and carried me along with them.

As the soiree came to a close, Vika, Maria, and Ivan braided their voices together in a final song. Beneath a canopy of stars, their eyes glistened with tenderness, and the girls' faces took on the texture of soft, creamy velvet. Their harmonies carried me back to the summers when they had serenaded Mike and me morning, noon, and night. The dance of love and affection flowing between Ivan and his daughters caused tears to well in my eyes. I had never experienced that dance with my father or with a child of my own, and never would. Sorrow still lingered from those losses. But now, on this starlit night in Vasilki, tears of grace and gratitude filled my soul with veins of gold.

Babushka's guests filled every nook in the house that night. To make room for everyone, Ivan and his friend slept outside in their cars. The house was quiet and Mike and I were about to crawl under the sheets when Babushka summoned us from the adjacent room. Already dressed for bed, we walked into the room and gasped. She was lying between two sheets on the still-warm clay oven, spilling over the sides of the narrow bridge between the dome and the wall. Smiling mischievously, Babushka closed her eyes. "*Spokoynoy nochi*," she said. *Good night.*

CHAPTER 25

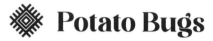 **Potato Bugs**

Ukraine

On the morning of our last day in the village, I rose quietly
and gently closed the bedroom door behind me. When I
looked up, I saw Babushka standing in the kitchen, towering
over a pot of water heating on the stove. She was wrapped
in a dress with wide hot-pink and black horizonal stripes,
with a green flowered scarf pulled tight across her forehead
and knotted at the nape of her neck, her bare feet covered
in dust.

"*Dobroye utro!*" she greeted me. *Good morning.* An
empty water bucket sat on the counter.

"*Dobroye utro!*" I replied. We were alone together for
the first time. Zoya and Ivan were back in Belarus. Ella
and Alex were in Vinnytsia. The girls were sleeping at
their cousins' house. There was no one around who could
translate, yet I felt comfortable alone with Babushka.

The early morning peace settled in around us. The sound
of a soft blue flame on the gas stove filled the silence. I felt
an unusual closeness to this colorful *babushka* I'd met just
two days earlier. Again, I ached with regret that I hadn't
learned her language. I longed to speak heart-to-heart with
this distiller of vodka who celebrated life with generosity

and humor despite the terrible tragedies she had endured. Just shy of seventy, she was a songbird of survival and mirth.

The intimacy of the moment carried the weight of knowing this could be our last visit. Though Babushka had joked about launching a new life in America with a pig in one arm and a boyfriend on the other, she was beginning to rust. The twins had told me she was troubled with heart problems and high blood pressure. As that reality seeped in, a sense of loss crept over me.

I thought about Babushka facing the quiet of a widow's life after Mike and I left with the twins that evening. Would that quiet bring her a sense of emptiness or welcome relief? Mike and I would soon return to an empty house and regular life as a family of two. The touch and voices of our global family would all too soon turn to memory, surreal like a dream.

Now, standing in the kitchen with the colorful grandmother, waiting for water to boil, I sensed the aura of sadness touched her too. Was she feeling sad for me? I thought about the Mary and Jesus icons she had sent to me one summer when the girls visited—"so you won't be sad when we leave."

I felt a tangle of emotions and a compelling urge to help Babushka in our last hours together. As a guest, I always wanted to pitch in. But this time, I would realize later, my genuine desire to help Babushka was tinged with guilt that stemmed from my ability to walk through life with privilege and ease.

"*Ya rabota*," I said. *I work.*

Pouring the heated water into two bowls, one for washing dishes, the other for rinsing, Babushka nodded knowingly. She washed and I dried in a comfortable silence. When all the dishes were stacked on shelves concealed behind a curtain, I thought we might sweep floors or dust furniture next.

But a different task was weighing on Babushka's mind. She motioned for me to follow her outside.

Curious, I traipsed behind her. At the edge of the potato field she stopped, snapped off the leafy top of a plant, and handed it to me. Every green leaf was etched with holes. I knew, from my early life on a farm, those holes could mean only one thing.

"Potato bugs!" I exclaimed. The summer of my seventh birthday, my dad had taught me how to protect our small plot of potatoes from total devastation by knocking the bugs off the leaves with a twig, into a tin can half filled with gasoline.

Certain I had grasped the situation, Babushka nodded. "*Da.*" Then she began growling and gnashing her teeth like a dog fighting for a bone, tossing her head from side to side, waving her arms from east to west. Stunning to behold, Babushka's performance of nonverbal communication made her point perfectly clear. The bugs would devour her entire crop if she didn't kill them quickly.

"*Da,*" I agreed. But I still couldn't imagine how I might help. There were far too many plants for two people to debug the way my father taught me. Our plot had been small, producing just enough potatoes to put on our table. Babushka's plants covered several acres. Most of her spuds were needed to fatten a pig for slaughter. The rest she used for cooking and for distilling vodka.

Reading my confusion, Babushka used her hands to mime a tubular shape about twelve inches in diameter and two feet high. She hoisted the imaginary tube onto her back and aimed her arm at the plants with fingers spread wide, like five streams diverging from a river.

My heart sank as it hit me. The invisible tube on Babushka's back represented a sprayer, her arm a hose, her fingers streams of poison. The deceptively sweet summer smell of pesticides sprayed on our farmland came rolling back to me. Alarms went off in my head. My mind raced. Babushka needed help spraying pesticides! Did she realize that breathing the toxic fumes could make her sick? Exposure to radiation from Chernobyl would have made her even more susceptible. Had exposure to radiation and pesticides triggered the heart condition and unexplained periods of illness she already suffered?

I desperately wanted to protect this woman, my adopted kin, as well as my own health. But there was no way I could explain to her the dangers of exposure to neurotoxins, hormone disruptors, and carcinogens. If I spoke her language, I could have warned her that the bugs would become resistant and require more and more costly chemicals, that farmers in India were committing suicide by drinking pesticides because the spiraling cost of increased resistance had left them destitute.

My mind jammed with words I couldn't unload. And I knew that even if I were able to communicate, it wouldn't make a difference. Babushka didn't have the option to farm organically. That method required time, money, energy, training, and other resources unavailable to her. If she didn't kill those potato bugs immediately, there would be no meat on her table that winter. Anxious to get on with the job, she pointed to the phantom tank on her back.

"Karina," she said, waving to me to follow her again. I understood that we would walk down the road to her daughter's house to get the tank.

"*Odin minuta. Ya* Mike," I said—shorthand for, "Just a minute, I'm going to let Mike know where we're going." Babushka nodded.

I sped into the house like a woman running from snakes. Mike was still sound asleep in bed. Birdsong drifted in through the open window.

"Mike, wake up!" I stage whispered. When he didn't respond, I touched his warm, dewy arm. "Mike!" His eyes blinked open. "Babushka wants me to spray the potato field with pesticides! We're going to Karina's right now to borrow the sprayer. What am I going to do?"

The words tumbled like an avalanche. My knight sat up in his boxers and planted his feet on the floor. "I'll do it," he croaked. "I'll dress while you and Babushka get the sprayer," he added, rubbing his eyes and finger-combing his short graying hair.

"I don't want you breathing those fumes either!"

"I'll wrap a T-shirt over my nose and mouth. I'll be okay."

"That won't protect you."

"We'll figure it out," he reassured me.

Babushka marched down the middle of the dirt road barefooted. Her cracked feet reminded me of a photograph I'd seen of Mother Teresa's knotty toes covered with dust and grime from the streets of Calcutta. Trying to keep up with Babushka, I stepped carefully, wearing good walking shoes, to avoid turning an ankle.

The houses we passed were distinguished mainly by their fences, each a different style and color, some with painted turned spindles. Later I would see these types of fences in a carnival of colors—yellow, blue, green, violet—surrounding Ukrainian cemeteries. We shared the road with roosters, a mama goose and her goslings, and barking dogs. Occasionally we crossed paths with an elder, slowly pumping the wheels of a rickety bicycle, a bundle strapped to their back and bags hanging from their handlebars. Fortunately, there were no cars on the road to kick up dust.

After rattling around the shed that sheltered Karina's cows, Babushka triumphantly lifted the sprayer and clung to it with determined satisfaction as we retraced our steps back to her house. The sun's heat wearied me. My clothes felt damp and sticky, my legs like seaweed. The humidity made me feel ill. Still, I was thankful there wasn't much of a breeze. That would keep the spray from drifting far.

Slowed by both heat and dread, I felt as though I were marching blindfolded toward a cliff. The sprayer dangled at Babushka's side. The grating of the attached hose dragging on the ground sounded like a warning. Danger! Poisons!

A frail old crone sat perched on an aging bench beside the road. Smiling, she patted the seat beside her as we approached. Weighing no more than a sack of potatoes, the sliver of a woman wore a dark long-sleeved blouse tucked into a skirt that dropped to her bird-like ankles, where her socks slumped into layers. Babushka greeted the lady but didn't pause to chat. She was on a mission. Wordlessly, she explained to her neighbor why she didn't have time to rest by raising the sprayer shoulder-high as we passed.

"*Da, da. Rabota, rabota, rabota,*" said the woman resting on the bench. *Yes, yes. Work, work, work.*

Babushka opened her gate, dropped the sprayer to the ground, plodded up to the porch, and disappeared inside the house. While I waited in the doorway, she reappeared with a little square of cardboard and carefully removed a small, attached capsule. Half green and half brown, it looked harmless. A stunning realization hit me: This was what chemical warfare looked like. That tiny pill the size of a Tylenol would contaminate the land for years. Itty-bitty capsules filled with neurotoxins could destroy all of civilization.

Holding the capsule, Babushka turned her head sideways and made a loud, forceful sound like it was shot from a cannon. "*Hooohhk!*" When I realized the blast of dry spit was Babushka's way of informing me that the innocent-looking capsule was toxic, I felt some relief. *Thank God she knows!*

Just as that message was delivered, Mike walked up. The detonation had startled him too, but he quickly regained his composure. He made motions as if he were putting invisible gloves on his hands. "Gloves? *Ya* gloves?" he asked Babushka.

When Babushka realized Mike intended to apply the chemicals, she scowled. *"Niet! Niet!"* She waved us toward the door as though pushing out intruders. *"Magazine! Khleb y syr!"* *Store. Bread and cheese.* She was sending us to the little village store to keep us out of harm's way while she sprayed the field.

"It's okay, I'll spray for you," Mike protested.

Babushka turned and left the room, mumbling under her breath. We could hear her rooting around in the back room. Baffled, I turned to Mike.

"What's she doing?"

"Maybe trying to find gloves for me?" Mike guessed. But he had underestimated Babushka's resolve.

When she returned, my jaw dropped. Wearing thick black leggings under an old work dress, a heavy sweater, and sturdy shoes, she looked like a Ukrainian version of the Tin Man from *The Wizard of Oz.*

"Magazine," she directed us again, hands on her hips. Once again, she had made her point clear. She alone would put herself in harm's way while Mike and I hoofed it to the market. Until then, she wouldn't budge.

A mixture of relief and guilt spun in my chest as Mike and I left through the gate and closed it behind us. Over our shoulders, we saw Babushka set off as though going to slay the Wicked Witch of the West. She wore no mask, no respirator, and no gloves. I wondered if the carcinogenic capsule clutched in her hand had been manufactured in the United States.

Years later I would see Babushka again, not in person but online, when Maria contacted me from Ukraine on

Skype. I was thrilled when she joined our conversation, though it felt strange to see her on my screen, sitting at a table enjoying a cup of tea. She looked much older and was missing teeth. To my surprise, she asked if I remembered that day when she sprayed the fields. Of course I did, I told her, wishing I knew what that event had meant to her. For me, her protection of Mike and me that day was an act of love.

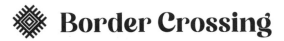 Border Crossing

Ukraine to Belarus

Sandwiched between the twins, I started down the long flight of wide, shallow stairs leading to an outdoor market across the street from the passenger railway station, Kyiv–Pasazhyrskyi. Maria was on the hunt for shoes to buy before we boarded the train to Belarus.

A dried-apple-faced woman wearing a widow's black dress stood on a landing in the blazing sun trying to eke out a living. She was holding little bunches of seeds wrapped in cloth and tied with string. *"Nasinnia soniashnyka?"* she asked. *Sunflower seeds?* On a mission and short on time, we didn't stop.

At the foot of the stairs, the horizon expanded to reveal a maze of stalls. Dizzied by the hot, dense air filled with scents of sweat, herbs, and strawberries spoiling in the sun, I felt my pulse quicken. Though I considered myself an aficionado of markets and had visited many in the United States, Mexico, and Western Europe, this one pulsed with a heavy vibe that triggered my apprehension. Picking up on my sudden tension, Vika clasped my hand like a mother hen and Maria took the lead through the crowded lanes. Twisting and turning, we sank deeper and deeper into a world of vendors selling imported clothes, CDs, jewelry, and household goods. Here and there, another weary widow in black peddled what little she could harvest from her garden. *Where are the local farmers? The street musicians? Artists selling handmade jewelry, paintings, handbags, and clothes?* They were the heart and soul of markets I was accustomed to and loved.

Maria darted from one vendor to another, searching for shoes as we wandered farther and farther away from the train station where we had left Mike guarding our bags. If we didn't return soon, he would worry. Thirsty, tired, and concerned about missing our train, I tried to hurry Maria.

"What about these?"

"*Niet.*"

"What about those?"

"*Niet.*"

"Maybe you don't buy shoes today," I said, feeling anxious. "It's almost time to board the train. We need to go."

Reluctantly, Maria turned to go back, and her mood soured. As we wound our way out of the convoluted market, she spotted footwear that suited her. She put the sandals on her feet and her mood instantly improved. After she made the purchase, we hurried through the crowd and up the stairs. As we crossed the street, I saw Mike, checking his watch.

"I shoes, Michael. You like?" Maria called to him, pointing to her feet.

"Yes, very nice. Now let's get going." His face looked pinched and nervous.

"Sorry. It took a bit longer than we expected," I said.

Throngs of people packed the station and waited outside to board trains headed to the Black Sea, Moscow, Warsaw, Budapest, Berlin, and beyond. In the confusion of people, tracks, signs, and announcements that baffled Mike and me, we were grateful to have the girls in the lead. Without a hitch, they delivered us to the aging blue train that would carry us to Belarus.

"I think attending school in Minsk has boosted the girls' confidence and made them street smart," I commented to Mike.

We had reserved two first-class compartments—one for us and one for the twins. Our side-by-side chambers were tidy and simple, with padded sleeping benches on each side of a table and curtains hung in the window. Maria and Vika stowed their bags and hurried off to visit two girls they knew, about their age, who worked on the train in the economy carriage. Traveling in first class, with Americans, qualified as big news, and they could hardly wait to tell their friends. Mike and I sat at our table, savoring a bottle of cold water and the drizzle of cool air that flowed through the vents.

"Are you ready for this?" Mike asked. I knew he was referring to crossing the border, when the train would stop in the middle of the night, deep in a forest near the exclusion zone of Chernobyl. Guards would board the train to question us and inspect our visas and passports.

"I'm ready!" The fear that had almost caused me to back out of the trip had lost its power.

"Good, because there's no turning back now!"

We were chugging across the underbelly of Kyiv when Vika and Maria slipped into our compartment, sidled in beside us, and closed the door.

Dark eyeliner enhanced Vika's steady gaze, first at Mike and then at me. "When we stop at border," she said, "say you have five hundred dollars." Her statement set my nerves on fire.

"We're not going to lie!" I blurted, unprepared for this conversation. Foreigners were allowed to bring up to fifteen hundred dollars into the country. I couldn't imagine why we would risk deceiving the border police.

"They will take some for themselves, Gail. We know this," Maria explained. "Say you have five hundred dollars," she repeated. Her blouse clung to her breasts and ribs. Color had been carefully applied to her eyelids. She was no longer the tomboy she'd been as a child. Vika's dark hair draped over her shoulders in sensual waves; coal-colored eyeliner accentuated the allure of her eyes.

"We can't say that!" I shot back. "They wouldn't believe us! We're Americans traveling in first class—they know we have more than that."

Our roles had been reversed. The girls were now our guides in a social, political, and cultural system where cooperating with corruption could be the price for survival. But I wasn't yet ready to trust their advice to lie to the border patrol. Nor was I prepared to acknowledge that they had been indoctrinated into a system of complex morals that I didn't understand.

To my horror, Mike began slipping money between the pages of his book. "What are you doing?" I screeched, shocked to see my trustworthy husband risk being caught in a lie that I feared could lead to our being detained or arrested at the border. When he didn't respond, my eyes darted from one side of our cabin to the other, searching for a hidden microphone or camera.

"I am telling the truth!" I said, in case anyone was listening.

Trying to make sense of the scene unfolding before me, I thought about the travel writer who had disabused me of my fear of being thrown into a Belarusian slammer. Now I wished I'd asked him what might happen to us if we were caught in a lie. It had never crossed my mind that I would need to know that kind of information.

Though the United States was not immune to corruption, it rarely intruded in my everyday life. It wouldn't have occurred to me that, all too soon, corruption would endanger the very pillars of democracy in the United States.

Now, with Mike's book fully loaded, he handed Maria and Vika each a fistful of bills. They buried the money inside their skimpy bras. Their low-cut blouses and lingerie revealed an abundance of skin and cleavage, but the cash had vanished completely. Intrigue danced in their eyes.

"We back soon!" Vika promised as she and Maria dashed off again to visit their friends.

"I think I'll take a look around. You wanna go with me?" Mike asked.

Still shocked, and hesitant to consort with a criminal, I shook my head no. Feeling as if I'd fallen down a rabbit hole into a strange new world, I puzzled over questions I hadn't considered before. *Did the girls find it necessary and normal to take money under false pretenses? Would they line their pockets with under-the-table money under certain circumstances? How would I feel if I knew they had done so? Would I exploit someone with deeper pockets than mine if I were in a desperate situation?*

I sat by the window watching miles of golden wheat fields and silvery birch forests streak by. The rural landscape and flashes of color soothed me. The train made occasional stops in villages where travelers were let on and off. Though I had no way of conversing with fellow passengers, I hungered to learn about their lives. Feeling isolated in first class, I ventured out hoping to at least rub elbows with the locals.

As the floor rocked beneath my feet, I made my first stop, in the lavatory. When I flushed the toilet, I could have sworn I saw the railroad tracks racing by through the hole that opened in the bottom of the toilet. To confirm, I flushed again. Blinded by my Western perspective of the world, I initially assumed this system for waste disposal existed only in undeveloped countries. Later, I learned it was still common practice all over the world and would take decades for direct-chute toilets to be replaced by holding tanks and compostable units.

With that discovery under my belt, I put a tinted gloss on my lips and made my way to the economy car. A blast of hot air, thick with the din of voices and scents of crowds and musty cheese, slapped my face when I opened the door. I saw passengers wiping sweat from the backs of their necks and above their lips. Some were already sleeping on the rows of slim wood benches attached to the walls, strangers snoring and snacking just inches from their faces. Feeling both guilt and gratitude, I returned to the comfort of our private compartment with its padded benches and cooled air.

At twilight, Mike and I enjoyed the simple supper of bread, cheese, and strawberries Babushka had sent with us. The girls joined us in our compartment, slurping on cups of instant soup they had purchased from a vending machine on board the train. I wouldn't have traded that moment, squished together around our table, enjoying our first meal alone together in years, for a candlelight dinner in a top-tier restaurant. While we talked, no one mentioned the border crossing.

"We show you where we take classes," said Maria.

"And Minsk," Vika added.

After dark, while the girls nested in their own compartment, I fluffed my pillow and changed into a T-shirt and comfortable shorts for sleeping. Mike camped on the bench across from me while I wrote in my journal, trying to assimilate the dream-like flow of the day's events. I fell asleep to the rocking of our carriage and slept peacefully until we reached the dark forest where the train groaned to a halt.

Wide-eyed, I sat up and turned on the light. As the train heaved into place, Mike, still fully dressed, sat up and slid open the door, ready to present our documents to the border police.

Though Mike would later tell me he had seen a small building with a light throwing shadows into the surrounding forest, I saw no lights, no buildings, no signs of life. Only blackness. A chill ran through me in the eerie stillness. *Will the guards search our belongings? Catch us in a lie? Will we be allowed to enter Lukashenko's domain?* Thinking of what might happen to someone removed from a train in this desolate place, I shuddered. In the distance, I heard the *whoosh* of a door opening, then footfalls.

Sleepy-eyed, Maria and Vika crawled in beside us to wait, ready to present their own documents and to translate for us. Their presence instilled in me a sense of belonging in this strange and unfamiliar place. The guards, Maria explained, would work their way through the economy cars first.

Knowing that on the narrow shelf behind me lay a book with fifty- and twenty-dollar bills hidden among its pages, and that the girls both had money stuck to their breasts, I felt surprisingly calm. Had my psyche created a kind of denial? Had I adopted a new moral code? Most likely, an overload of adrenaline prevented me from feeling much of anything. The fight, flight, or freeze mechanism had taken over, and I froze.

With another *whoosh*, the door into our carriage opened, and I heard the deep, monotone voice of a guard. With my heart thumping hard, I scanned Mike and the girls for subtle nuances that might convey their culpability as we waited in silence. All three looked impassive and bored, like teenagers forced to ride in a car with their mother.

Suddenly, two guards were standing over us. Expecting hard-faced hulks, I felt my jaw drop when I saw their faces. They were boys. Though they seemed too young to shave, they were armed with an air of authority and rifles strapped across their chests. Their tall hats created an illusion of height. These were the faces of soldiers everywhere, through all of time, I realized.

One guard appeared disinterested and didn't speak. The other one spoke without making eye contact. His voice was clipped.

"Your documents," Vika translated.

Mike handed him both of our passports, a bit too eagerly, I thought. The young man opened Mike's first, studied it briefly, then asked how much money he was bringing into the country. I held my breath.

"Eight hundred dollars," Mike answered in a calm and even voice. The girls didn't blink an eye.

When the guard reached for my passport, I imagined the book that lay on a shelf less than a foot away from me was flashing like a red light he couldn't help but notice. Fortunately, it was behind me, where I wouldn't accidentally look at it and tip him off. *Is there money sticking out between the pages?* Without looking at me or the book, the guard asked how much money I was carrying.

"Fifteen hundred dollars."

The young man's back stiffened. Alarm flashed across his face. Not fluent in English, he had misunderstood me. "Fifteen thousand dollars?" His voice had dropped an octave.

"No! One thousand five hundred dollars!" I sputtered, my heart pounding as Vika translated. *How could this happen? I'm the one telling the truth, and I'm the one who's going to be arrested!*

The guard's back relaxed again. Without another word to Mike or me, he handed back our passports and turned his attention to the girls. I tried to breathe normally, though I knew we wouldn't be out of the woods until he finished with Vika and Maria. A shudder ripped through me when I saw the guard's eyes roam to their bosoms. The glance he stole was so quick that I knew it was for his own pleasure, not motivated by suspicion. I didn't want an armed man ogling my girls for any reason, but I was in no position to express my opinions.

Though our interaction with the guards had lasted under five minutes, my muscles felt wobbly, like I'd been lifting weights for hours. When the guards returned to their post in the forest, my heart started to slow as the great blue train rolled across the border.

Mike and I slapped hands in a high-five. "We're in Belarus!" I whooped.

At daybreak, I popped out of bed and stood at a window in the corridor to capture my first glimpse of the country. A coral horizon greeted me. Wisps of fog hovered over ponds and bogs. Trees and crops in every shade of green, from emerald to chartreuse, rolled by. It was the time of year when tractors plowing fields and planting crops kicked up radiation in the soil. I prayed that invisible risk wouldn't impact my health, already compromised by pesticides and other chemicals.

Despite the risk, reaching Belarus was for me a holy moment. I knew that only love could have coaxed me here and disarmed the legacy of Cold War fears instilled in me as a child. I could feel the loose threads of my life coming together as I stood watching the sunrise, trying to feel the soul of a place with deep connections for me, memorizing its tapestry.

Maria broke my trance when, half awake, she emerged from her compartment. "Good morning, Gail. Soon we stop. You say to Mike bring bags to door. Papa wait for us. Train stop three minutes only. We must get off quickly."

A bolt of excitement shot through me. When I delivered Maria's message, Mike was up and dressed but still a bit foggy.

"We're almost at the stop where Ivan's picking us up! Maria said we need to hurry. The train stops for only three minutes."

I quickly changed into my clothes, stuffed my journal and sleeping attire into my bag, ran my fingers through my hair, and headed toward the exit door pushing my roller bag, a second bag swinging from my shoulder.

"I'm right behind you," Mike assured me.

We joined the girls with just moments to spare. With no building or platform in sight, the train slowed to a halt with a painful screech. When the doors opened, I saw only one person: Ivan, in his black slacks and a short-sleeved summer shirt, jogging toward us across patchy grassland dotted with wildflowers and butterflies, to muscle our bags to the car. Overflowing with excitement, curiosity, and awe, I hustled down the steps behind the girls while Mike tossed a bag to Ivan. Standing on Belarusian soil for the first time, I felt an urge to dance. I twirled halfway around just in time to see *moy muzh Misha*—my husband Michael—leap from the train.

CHAPTER 27

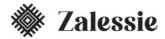 **Zalessie**

Belarus

Strong and muscular from physical labor, Ivan easily hoisted our bags into the trunk of his car, a small, older model he tinkered with regularly to keep in good running condition. Though he wasn't one to show a lot of emotion, his peaceful smile, bright eyes, and relaxed jaw conveyed a warm welcome. As he drove the girls and us to their apartment in Zalessie, he rested his tanned arm, bent at the elbow, on the open window.

A cloud of dust followed us as we sped along a bumpy unpaved road across a landscape of farmland. The flat terrain, earthy smell, and wheat fields carried me back to my roots. Even the sound of tires on gravel and the trail of dust behind us struck a familiar chord. But the fields stretched beyond the size of any I saw growing up. And, I didn't see farmhouses or barns, as I was accustomed to seeing in the United States.

Eager to introduce us to their way of life in Belarus, Ivan explained that the state owned and operated most of the land; the men who worked these vast parcels, including him, were government employees who lived in villages. The twins translated his commentary the best they could with their limited English.

"Central base," Ivan said, pointing with his chin toward a nondescript building. It was where the state-owned farm machinery was stored and repaired, Vika explained. The tractors and equipment I could see behind the concrete fence surrounding the property struck me as surprisingly large and modern for a poor country.

A minute later I noticed a vehicle coming toward us from the opposite direction, and I realized it was a horse-drawn wagon. Ivan tried to explain that strange juxtaposition, but the twins found the concept difficult to translate. If I understood correctly, the man with the wagon was a collective farmer, someone who leased land on a state-owned farm that had been divided into small parcels. Collective farmers, I read later, commonly relied on their own manual labor and horse-drawn plows and wagons because tractors were not affordable for solo farmers. The disparity seemed extreme.

The only people I knew of who might still farm with horses in the United States were the Mennonites and Amish, who rejected modernity for religious purposes. Even back in the 1950s, when my parents had struggled to make ends meet, my dad had always owned his own tractors and other equipment. When he gave up farming, he improved our standard of living by selling the land, moving to a city, and working in an automobile factory as a machine repairman. Though he wasn't cut out for city life, he made that choice because it would provide health insurance for our family and a steady income that enabled my siblings and me to attend college. I wondered if the farmers in Belarus had options.

When Ivan drove into a village of four-story Soviet-style buildings, I knew we had arrived in Zalessie. I recognized the bland apartment buildings from pictures I'd seen of the girls playing outside in the snow.

"This day care and school," said Vika, pointing to a nearby building with a small playground.

"Is that where you and Maria went to school?"

"*Da.*"

Ivan parked near the building where they lived. We unloaded the bags and walked toward the entrance, a metal door with a window covered by a metal grid. I felt as if we were headed into a high-security building where secret documents were stored. A tangle of curiosity and caution caught in my chest. Then Maria pointed up, and I recognized Zoya eagerly waving to us from a window. Sensing her excitement put me at ease.

Holding our largest bag with one hand, Ivan held the door open for the rest of us. Climbing the concrete stairwell with two of the smaller bags, I sniffed the air, hoping I wouldn't detect scented laundry products or other chemicals that made me ill. I never knew when I might be hit with exposures, especially in multifamily buildings where scents could drift from under the doors of other dwellings. So far, I'd been lucky on this trip. At Babushka's, I realized none of the men, including Ivan, wore aftershave or other strong-smelling products, and none of the women wore perfume. I didn't know if that was typical or if they'd been informed that fragrances could make me sick. Now, when I realized the air in the stairwell smelled fresh, I took a deep breath of relief.

Waiting at the top of the stairs to greet us with her bright smile and easygoing manner, Zoya stood in the doorway of their apartment. Dressed in a casual tropical-print dress with bright pink flowers against a sea-blue background, her short brown hair perfectly in place, she looked perky despite staying up late to confirm we'd had no trouble crossing the border.

"Michael! Gail!" said Zoya, making room for us to carry our bags across the threshold.

After years of sending and receiving cards and letters to and from this address, I took my first step inside the cozy one-bedroom apartment where Zoya and Ivan had raised their three daughters. I caught a hint of a savory scent drifting from the kitchen. Flooded with a combination of excitement, curiosity, nerves, and disbelief, my heartbeat quickened.

We entered a narrow hallway. Cupboards and coats hanging from hooks covered the wall on our left. While we paused there to remove our shoes, the Nervous Nellie part of me felt a moment of panic. *This is going to be awkward!*

It wasn't as if we were meeting Zoya and Ivan for the first time, of course. But this would be our first time spending days together and sleeping under the same roof without the bright light of Babushka's presence. In Ukraine, I had the impression that Zoya was slightly shy, like me. Ivan had struck me as a man of few words who gladly worked behind the scenes to host us and our friends. Mike could strike up a conversation with most anyone—in English—but the language barrier had made him feel awkward in social situations. In Babushka's absence, it would take all of us to light up the room.

Fortunately, my wiser self was reassuring. *You've known and loved these twins for ten years. You've been waiting for this moment to experience their world, and now it's here. You're feeling what they must have felt the first time they came to stay with you when they were only eight years old. Let the magic unfold, just as they did!*

To the right, behind French doors, was a long rectangular room illuminated by light coming through a window at the far end. Sheer curtains and opened drapes adorned with gold spirals dressed the window from floor to ceiling. I caught glimpses of a sofa, a television, a buffet, and a rug hanging on one wall—just as I had seen at Babushka's. The sight of Ivan's forest-green accordion sitting on the floor rekindled the deep satisfaction I felt in Ukraine when he had squeezed its bellows and played its keys. Excitement fluttered in my chest. *Maybe he'll play for us again!*

"This way," said Maria, leading us down the hallway to the bedroom she and Vika shared, on the left at the end of the hall.

The first thing I saw when we stepped into the room were stuffed bears sitting on the gold satin bedspread; I remembered the girls buying those bears at yard sales in Seattle, when we went bargain hunting on Saturday mornings. Then my eyes darted to birthday cards we'd sent to them, standing on a shelf at the head of the bed. Seeing those totems of our history together, and realizing they had kept them close, nearly brought me to tears and told me I was exactly where I belonged.

"You and Mike sleep here," stated Vika.

"But where will you sleep?"

"We sleep in room with Mama and Papa." The back of the sofa I'd seen in the living room folded flat to make a bed. Ivan and Zoya always slept there, leaving the bedroom for their daughters.

The thought of sleeping in a private bedroom while the rest of the family slept on the floor and sofa made me uncomfortable. Yet I didn't want to make an awkward fuss, so I didn't protest. But Maria read my face.

"It's okay, Gail," she assured me. "No problem."

Through a door across the room, Vika ushered us out to a porch, five by eight feet, enclosed with sheets of plastic. A wood-framed window swung out over an expansive view of green and gold fields and a village on the horizon.

"What a beautiful view!" Mike remarked.

"Papa smoke cigarettes here," said Vika, pointing to the open window. Smoking wasn't allowed in the rest of the apartment. Later I would learn that it was customary to keep windows closed to prevent illness caused by a direct breeze coming in from the outside, even during the summer. I didn't ask why the porch window was an exception; I concluded it was because, technically, the porch was outdoors, separated from the apartment by a door that blocked the breeze from drifting inside.

"When warm outside, we put clothes here to dry," said Maria.

Vika pointed to a collection of canning jars filled with pickles and salads sitting in a corner. "Mama make with food from *dacha*."

After hearing about the *dacha* from the girls and in letters Zoya wrote to us over the years, the farm girl in me had always wanted to go there. Though *dachas* had acquired a romantic history as rural second homes of noblemen, the term now also applied to humble garden plots owned by common people, with or without some kind of shack or cottage where they could spend the night in the country.

Zoya suggested we nap for a couple hours before she served breakfast. "First, show them where to use the toilet and sink," she instructed Maria.

Maria pointed toward two doors sandwiched between the bedroom and kitchen. Hidden behind one door was a small cubicle furnished with a toilet. The second door opened into a room large enough to accommodate a small vanity with a sink, a bathtub with a shower, and a water tank. Fresh towels lay on the vanity.

As I washed my hands and face, I imagined Zoya scrubbing laundry at the sink or on her knees beside the tub, then hanging everything over the tub to dry when the porch was too damp or cold. I knew this was common practice throughout Europe and many other countries and had washed my own clothes by hand when traveling. But this was the first time it fully registered in my brain how difficult it was to *always* have to wash every towel, tablecloth, sheet, sock, and each stitch of clothing by hand for a family. No wonder they kept their wardrobes to a minimum! I flashed back to the one little black duffel the girls brought to Seattle each summer, and the house in Ukraine where all the clothes we'd sent home with them were stored. Now it all made perfect sense and it brought home to me, again, that life in the United States had distorted my view of how much *stuff* is "enough."

After a refreshing nap, Mike and I joined the family in the compact and welcoming kitchen, where beautiful white sheer curtains with tassels as long as my arms hung in a large window. Zoya stood in front of a four-burner stove pouring batter into a skillet.

"*Bliny*," she said.

Potted plants sat on the wide sill, thriving in the sun. Through the window, I could see all the buildings connected by pathways and facing a grassy common area. The only sign of life I saw outside, that early in the morning, were finches sitting in the branches of a tree near the window. Zoya told us that, earlier, the birds had sat right up next to the glass, on a narrow ledge, signaling the imminent arrival of guests. Smiling as I pictured the little birds assuring her that we were on our way, I had the sense that Zoya and I might be cut from the same cloth.

Ivan directed Mike and me to sit on a cushioned bench along one side of a small table in the corner. Zoya delivered the *bliny*, sour cream, jelly, and cartons of juice to the table, then she and Ivan sat on round wood stools across from us. Maria and Vika sat on stools they placed at the end of the table opposite the window. Without the extended family present, there was enough calm and quiet to have our first real conversation.

"How did you and Ivan meet?" I asked Zoya.

They were both Ukrainians, she said. They met in a village in Ukraine, near Chernobyl, where both families had lived. After the evacuation, she and Ivan were the only members of their families to leave Ukraine.

"Why didn't you go with the rest of your family?" asked Mike.

"We saw more opportunity here," replied Ivan. "At that time, Belarus was part of the Soviet Union, like Ukraine."

"It was difficult to separate from our families," added Zoya. "But the apartments they built for us here had hot and cold running water and a flush toilet, modern conveniences we'd never had and would not have had we relocated in Ukraine."

"What's the current population of Zalessie?" Mike asked.

"About five thousand."

"We have a grocery store, bus transportation, and a few small stores," said Zoya, pouring instant coffee.

"Have you been working in agriculture since you got here?" Mike asked Ivan.

"No, I still worked at Chernobyl when we came to Zalessie. After the explosion, I was part of a crew of liquidators who cleaned up the debris. We worked in shifts, two weeks on and two off." I thought I saw a hint of grief in his gray-blue eyes. The effects of his exposure to radiation were not yet visible.

Although I knew that Ivan had worked as a liquidator, for some inexplicable reason it didn't seem possible to be sitting across the table from him, talking about it face-to-face, as matter-of-factly as if we were discussing the weather. I couldn't imagine what must have gone through his mind while he performed the work that machines couldn't do because they had been disabled by the radiation.

"How did you feel about working as a liquidator?" I asked.

"It had to be done. You just did what you had to do. And we drank vodka!" he added with an ironic laugh, flashing a warm smile and his gold tooth. In his eyes, I saw a gentle soul who kept the trials and tribulations he had faced locked deep inside.

An awkward pause followed that comment. I wanted to blurt out what we'd heard in the United States—that the Soviets advised the liquidators to drink vodka to "kill" the radiation they absorbed and didn't provide them with protective clothing or masks. But this was not the time or the place for my views from the West.

"And then you girls were born!" said Mike, steering the conversation in a different direction.

"*Da!*" Zoya smiled.

"When you were pregnant with the twins, were you worried they might be impacted by radiation?" I asked. Without thinking about it first, I had circled back to the topic of Chernobyl, despite Mike's efforts.

"Oh no," Zoya answered. "The explosion happened two years before they were born. We didn't need to worry about that."

Stunned, I didn't know how to respond. Our views of the dangers posed by radiation were vastly different. I felt uneasy, as though I had stepped into a dissonant reality, where opposing information must remain unexamined in order to carry on with daily life. My mind spun with questions. *How had the purpose of the Children of Chernobyl program been explained to her? Did she or Ivan question the accuracy of information provided by the Soviets? Were they informed that more than 60 percent of the nuclear fallout had landed in Belarus, and some of it would take hundreds of years or more to break down?*

Not wanting to address those politically sensitive issues,

I didn't ask any of the questions burning in me. Our conversation ended there with the arrival of the twins' sister, Elina, her husband Sergey, and their baby girl for a second seating at the breakfast table. The terrible explosion that had brought us together was never mentioned again.

"Gail! Mike! Hello!" they greeted us in English. Their warm hugs conveyed they were as happy to finally meet as I was.

Elina was a blonde, fair-skinned woman who, unlike Maria and Vika, wore no makeup. I knew she had been troubled by health issues since her exposure to radiation as a toddler. Now, dressed in a bright pink sleeveless top and denim jeans, she looked radiant. I'd heard so much about her through the years, I felt like I knew her already.

Towering over Elina, Sergey held six-month-old Liya against his shoulder, patting her back. A construction worker and former paratrooper with a rugged face and a scar on his cheek, his engaging personality and tenderness quickly endeared him to me.

In her Russian father's muscular arms, Liya looked extremely tiny but not at all frail. Holding her head high, she fixed her bright blue eyes on us with studied interest and came to me without hesitation when I held my arms out to her.

"You look ready to embrace the world," I cooed to her, wondering what the future held for this beautiful girl, the first granddaughter in this resilient family of Chernobyl survivors.

Later, I was thrilled when Zoya asked if we'd like to visit the *dacha*.

"I'd love to!" I answered.

Elina, Sergey, and Vika volunteered to stay home so the rest of us would fit into Ivan's car. "We'll take the baby with us," offered Zoya.

Ivan drove us out into the country and turned onto a gravel drive with a sign hung on an arch overhead. It said CORNY. *Roots.* The only buildings in sight were a small gray house and a barn, both with corrugated tin roofs. The house appeared vacant and leaned slightly, as though life had sucked the air out of it. I didn't see any cultivated areas until Ivan parked on the edge of the two-track road, alongside their land in this community of *dachas.*

There were no buildings on their property yet, not even a driveway. Just row after row of green plants reaching for the sun on a piece of earth bigger than a "P-Patch" in Seattle's community gardens and smaller than a baseball field. Enough to provide an escape from the confines of apartment life, an intimate connection to nature, an abundance of food in times of shortages, and a sense of ownership and freedom. I got the impression this place felt more like home to Ivan and Zoya than Zalessie.

"It's beautiful!" I remarked. They smiled proudly.

"Is a lot of work," grumbled Maria. She explained that it was a full-time job that began in the fall when they dried seeds from their harvest. In the early spring, they planted the seeds in paper cups to grow starts inside. As soon as the weather warmed up, Ivan furrowed and tilled the land, and the starts were put in the ground. Summer weekends and evenings were devoted to weeding and watering. After the fall harvest, Zoya made the salads and pickles they would eat through the winter. Then the cycle began again.

Zoya walked in front of me with Liya in her arms as we strolled up and down the furrows, admiring a panoply of vegetable plants. Cabbage and cucumbers. Tomatoes and beets. Potatoes and carrots. Peeking over Zoya's shoulder, the baby, dressed in a lime green triangle scarf and matching jumper, studied me with big, round eyes. On a miniature pesticide-free farm, surrounded by people I loved, serenaded by birds in nearby trees, I was in my happy place.

"Are these onions over here?" I asked Maria.

"*Da.*"

"And dill!"

"*Da,*" she said, breaking off a feathery leaf and popping it into her mouth.

By the time we left the *dacha*, images of that hallowed place were tattooed on my heart.

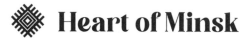 Heart of Minsk

Belarus

Russian pop music blared from the radio as we headed to Minsk in a van with Vika, Maria, Elina, and Sergey. Though sixteen years had passed since the fall of the Soviet Union, the city was still known for human rights restrictions and a heavy police presence. I half expected to see goose-stepping soldiers patrolling the streets.

Beaming with pride, Vika waved a red-and-green Belarus flag the size of a paperback book as we zipped along the highway. Elina's friend Vlad, our driver and the owner of the van, parked in the heart of the city.

Unlike the hustle and bustle of Kyiv, Minsk, a city of two million people, had a calm and orderly presence. I didn't see a single blemish of litter or graffiti. There was plenty of traffic, but no speeding, double parking, blasting horns, or squealing brakes.

Maintaining a steady clip, long-legged Sergey took the lead on our walk through the city. Vika walked beside me, her every step broadcasting confidence. Her sweet turned-up nose and the way her feet owned the pavement told me she understood the terms of navigation in a culture of which I knew so little. She felt safe. She belonged.

Immersing myself in the twins' world for the first time, this was a victory walk for me. Giddy with delight, I was behind the Iron Curtain at last.

I searched the faces of the steady stream of pedestrians, curious about the differences in ethnic diversity in this part of the world. In Seattle, the majority of the population claimed northern European descent. But I was also accustomed to seeing Asians, Latinos, African Americans, Indians, and Native Americans who lived there. Besides Belarusians and Ukrainians, Minsk was home to Russians, Poles, and many smaller minorities, but their various skin tones and other ethnic differences were almost indistinguishable to my American eyes.

Chiseled buildings greeted us at every turn like fortresses in shades of gray, reflecting Joseph Stalin's reconstruction of Minsk after it was decimated in World War II. One exception was a twenty-three-story glass structure shaped like a diamond set on a pedestal.

"National Library Belarus," said Sergey, pointing to the city's new architectural triumph sparkling in the distance. Reflecting the sky, it was an azure gem floating in a sea of gray. A beacon of change in a country where the state still owned and censored the media. Later I would learn that non-VIP residents weren't allowed access to some of the books on its shelves.

"Is beautiful, yes, Gail?" asked Maria, tossing her blonde hair behind her shoulder. Her navel peeked out between a spaghetti-strapped camisole and a silver-buckled leather belt attached to a black miniskirt. Remembering her as the child who never brushed her hair, I was still shocked to see her taking ownership of her feminine beauty and power.

"*Krasivaya!*" I agreed.

The award-winning design was a rhombicuboctahedron, a stunning conglomerate of eight triangles, six squares, and twelve rectangles. Glittering and calm as the river it faced, its features were both brawny and sensual. The feminine in Minsk was subtle. A curve in the road. A meandering river. A bare shoulder.

As we followed Sergey across the city, Mike stopped frequently to decipher signs and study street names. I had some concern he might get left behind until I realized that Vlad kept his eyes on us at all times. The wiry young man with a shaved head and thick black eyebrows, dressed entirely in black, halted in his tracks the moment Mike or I strayed or stopped and didn't budge until we rejoined the pack. Regardless of our pace, he remained approximately ten steps behind us, constantly talking on his cell phone. *Is he watching out for us so we don't get lost? Could he be tracking and reporting our whereabouts to government officials?*

"Maybe he's part of the KGB!" I whispered to Mike, only half jesting. Mike responded to my remark with raised eyebrows and a nonverbal warning that said, *Zip it, Gail!*

Years later, I told my Ukrainian friend Ella about my suspicions. "No," Ella responded. "Vlad talking to friends. Very unusual to have American visitors. He's telling friends what's going on."

While Vlad tracked us, I kept an eye out for coffee houses, stores with interesting window displays, and street markets. Those were the kinds of places where I usually acquired a sense of the personality and creativity of cities I visited. But not in Minsk, as it turned out. I didn't see coffee houses or window displays. One department store we saw was dominated by a massive gray sculpture, the *Heroic Soviet*, hanging above the entrance. This landmark, like the many war memorials in Minsk, reinforced the archetype of strength and sacrifice embodied by the culture, an all-for-one-and-one-for-all way of thinking.

I encountered no street vendors selling stuffed cabbage

rolls or other treats. No musicians busking for rubles. And only one artist—a student sitting and sketching at the top of a staircase near an art school. *Where are all the artists?* I wondered. In Seattle, artists, food vendors, musicians, farmers, fishermen, and sometimes even poets conducted business in public squares and markets. Finally it dawned on me, that was a difference between a consumer-driven, free-enterprise economy and a post-Soviet, highly central-ized system.

I was also surprised that I didn't see anyone in Minsk who appeared to be homeless. In Seattle, there were thou-sands of adults and children with no roof over their heads. Many of them suffered from drug and alcohol addiction and mental illness. Others worked but weren't paid enough to cover the expenses of renting an apartment or buying a house. Some slept in shelters provided by the city. Hundreds slept in parks and doorways and stood on street corners and freeway exits begging for money. *Does everyone in Minsk have a roof over their head?* I wondered. That didn't seem possible. Belarus was less than twenty years removed from the scarcity of food and basic essentials that was pervasive before the fall of the Soviet Union. Austerity still seemed prevalent. *Are homeless people in Minsk kept hidden or jailed?* Later, Maria confirmed that they existed, but she was vague about where they were and how they lived.

Finally, we reached our destination, the Holy Spirit Cathedral, an ancient treasure of Minsk where the Petrovy family prayed in times of need and celebration. Sergey, broad-chested and muscular, stood like a granite sculpture of Slavic strength in the foreground of the snowy-white Orthodox shrine. Flanked by a fresco of Mother Mary between the cathedral's two towers, he and the Holy Mother created a juxtaposition that represented wholeness to me, a potent melding of masculine and feminine.

Women were required to cover their heads to enter the sanctuary. When Elina purchased three headscarves at a kiosk and handed them to the twins and me, I asked, "Don't you want one for yourself?" Wearing her signature denim jeans and sleeveless pink blouse, she glanced away, but I could still see the tears nesting in her eyes.

"*Niet*."

Muddled by confusion, I turned to Maria.

"Since Elina lost baby, she not go to church." Maria's eyes were filled with sadness too.

I knew that Elina's first pregnancy had ended with the death of her baby, a boy, during her third trimester. Now the mother of a healthy six-month-old girl, she had seemed resilient, but at this moment I saw that her grief was still raw. I touched the soft flesh of her arm.

"I'm so sorry," I said softly, knowing there were no words that could ease the pain.

In the sanctuary, smoke and incense hung in the air. Dim light emanated from ornate chandeliers and cast shadows around the room. A shudder ran through me. Dark corners seemed to speak of the painful past, when Vladimir Lenin, a founder of the Communist party, had banned all religious services, stripped the sacred icons from the walls, and used the cathedral as a gymnasium and prison.

Like moths to a flame, the twins and I were drawn to the prayer candles burning on the altar table. There, as we lit candles and stood in the soft amber light and dancing shadows, my heart cracked open. I thought about Elina's tragic loss. Her exposure to radiation as a baby. The chronic health issues that had plagued her childhood. *Had radiation exposure caused her baby's death? Did she blame God? How many generations would be affected by Chernobyl?* I prayed for Elina and all mothers who had lost children.

Maria leaned into me. Vika stood on her other side. The illumination of the girls' faces filled me with warmth. As we watched our prayers burn against the dark, peace descended on me. I remembered feeling the same peace at the Taizé service I had attended with the girls in Seattle, the night I had prayed my bond with Maria and Vika would never break. Now, standing together on holy ground, I knew my prayer had been answered.

We left the sanctuary while our flames still flickered. Elina greeted us with a wistful smile. The twins and I removed our headscarves as we all followed Sergey along the River Svislach to the Isle of Tears, a tiny island built to commemorate the Belarusian soldiers killed in the Soviet-Afghan War.

On the Isle of Tears stood a small chapel surrounded by haunting metal statues of women draped in robes and veils like black Madonnas. Their hands held empty bowls and pictures of loved ones whose lives had been cut short by war. Steeped in death, the grieving women represented the mothers, wives, grandmothers, sisters, aunts, and lovers left behind. The anguish emanating from them expressed the sorrow carried by women on every continent. Grief permeated the air.

I, too, was a sister left behind by a brother—a brother who would have gone to war in Vietnam if melanoma hadn't claimed him first. I was a grieving mother without a child. I grieved that the weapons used by the Taliban, to kill Soviets, had been supplied by the United States. And I grieved that our countries' leaders still resorted to sending young men and women to die in senseless wars.

A cool, soft breeze floated across the slow-moving river. Standing under an arch of the chapel, I reached up and touched the face of one grieving woman. Though made of metal, it felt soft and smooth, like skin warmed by the sun.

In her sad eyes and gaunt cheeks, I saw the depths of suffering and found solace in the universal language of loss. There, in the city where I had seen remnants of the Iron Curtain, I knew I was looking at the feminine face of God.

CHAPTER 29

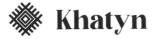 **Khatyn**

Belarus

The Khatyn State Memorial Complex was impossible to describe with a few words of English, so the twins arranged for a family friend to go with us and tell its chilling story to Mike and me in our language. Mike and I were familiar with the lovely young woman, Yulia, a former Children of Chernobyl participant who was just beginning a career as a translator.

Thirty miles outside of Minsk, the expansive complex was surrounded by birch trees and wildflowers. Despite its resemblance to a tranquil park with statuary and walking paths, it was a haunting place built by the Soviets to honor the Belarusian people and villages slaughtered during the German occupation in World War II.

Maria and I looped arms after we spilled out of Vlad's van. As we stood near the entrance to the grounds we heard a mournful sound, like a ghost crying for help. My heart lurched. Maria leaned into me and Vika's eyes opened wide.

"Bells," Mike said, pointing. We all turned. In the distance, there were more than two dozen bell towers. Each one stood on a square of earth the size of a small garden outlined with concrete curbs.

"One bell rings every thirty seconds, to represent how quickly Belarusians were killed during the German occupation," explained Yulia. "Each one marks a house that once stood here, in the village of Khatyn, before they were all burned to the ground. This skeleton village represents thousands of villages that were destroyed."

Slowly, we moved toward the site of the former village as if we were walking in a funeral procession. When another bell rang out like a wailing mother, I realized we were at ground zero for the grief that scars the soul of Belarus.

I shuddered when Yulia explained that the villagers had been locked in barns and burned alive, most of them women, infants, children, and elders. This was the closest I had ever come to standing in a death camp, and I couldn't track all that I was hearing and feeling. I sensed the presence of some dimension I couldn't name, as though souls of the slaughtered villagers were floating around us, trying to convey a message.

A sudden breeze lifted strands of Yulia's long dark hair. Calm and poised, she brushed a strand away from her face and continued the story. "Over two million people died in the war in our small country during the three-year occupation. Almost one-quarter of the population!" she emphasized. I couldn't imagine one of every four US citizens dying that way.

As I followed our young chaperones through the complex of shrines, our steps slowed to a crawl. Fingers of loss and trauma seemed to tighten around my throat. As we stood speechless in front of a towering statue of the only adult survivor of Khatyn, with his dead son draped across his arms, Mike broke the silence.

"It's hard to believe that the people who did this were young people like you, young German soldiers," he said, standing beside Sergey.

Sergey, who had served in the Russian military, turned to Mike. "No! *Germans* not do this. *Fascists* do this!" he said emphatically. World War II had ended long before Sergey's birth, but the passion he expressed felt fresh and raw.

At that time, I didn't know how to interpret his comment. Weren't the German soldiers Nazis, and weren't the Nazis fascists? There was so much I wanted to know and, regretfully, didn't question. It felt like too much to ask, given the language barrier and complexity of the issues. And I was just beginning to recognize fascist views in my own country, and the divisions they can create in families and communities.

Troubled by all this, I followed up with research after I returned to Seattle. I learned the special battalion responsible for the massacre at Khatyn included not only Germans but also Ukrainian nationalists and other Soviets who collaborated with the Nazis out of self-preservation or anti-communist sentiments. I wondered, then, if Sergey's emotion reflected the pain and anger of betrayal those villagers must have felt when fellow Soviets turned against them. And I realized his remark had pointed to important truths: that not all German soldiers were fascists and not all fascists were German.

In my search for answers, I stumbled upon a disturbing assertion that the size and emotional charge of the Khatyn memorial complex were designed to blur the significance of a place with a similar name—Hatyn—where the Soviets had murdered more than twenty thousand Polish prisoners of war. As much as that information jarred me, it made me pause to remember the distorted narratives and cover-ups in my own country, where history textbooks were fraught with oversimplification and hidden truths. The attempted genocide of Native Americans wasn't taught in schools when I received my education. The atrocities of slavery were consistently minimized. The ongoing murder of Black Americans and other people of color by law enforcement officers and white civilians was rationalized. Wounded Knee, the Tulsa race massacre, and other mass killings on US soil were whitewashed.

Khatyn was a haunting reminder of the atrocities of human violence against other humans everywhere. We left in a somber mood, each of us wrangling with the intrusive past and complex truths.

As we drove back to Zalessie, quiet filled the van like tea steeping in a cup. My thoughts and feelings kaleido-scoped from inexplicable horror to the miracle of the present moment. Through the unlikely portal of a nuclear explosion, Mike and I—Americans from the Cold War generation—had been brought together with this group of young people in the former Soviet Union. We were growing relationships from seeds of curiosity and compassion, and we had reached across the divides of our four nations—Russia, Ukraine, Belarus, and the United States—to stand together with endless knots of convoluted history and shifting alliances beneath our feet.

I glanced at Maria over my shoulder. She caught my eye with a warm smile. When I turned forward again, Vlad and I locked eyes for a brief but connected encounter in the rearview mirror. I felt a sense of wonder and belonging in our troupe of kindred souls.

Ten years later I would recognize the terrifying face of fascism in the United States and hear its rhetoric spoken by our own president, and many who supported him. His racist comments and aggressive effort to undermine the legitimacy of journalism, science, and the electoral process would threaten our democracy and send chills down my spine. As I watched the divides in politics and race deepen in my homeland, I thought I finally understood what the ghosts of Khatyn had tried to impress upon me: Humankind's only hope is for us to engage our so-called enemies with curiosity and compassion instead of hatred and greed.

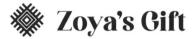 **Zoya's Gift**

Belarus

Ivan greeted us at the top of the stairwell when we returned from our tour. Straddled on his hip, six-month-old Liya gurgled with excitement and waved her arms to and fro. Scents of dough, herbs, and broth drifted from the kitchen into the hall and pulled us through the open door.

The living room had been transformed by the addition of a long table covered with a gold cloth. Set for a dinner party, it held shot glasses, vodka, a trio of salads, and platters holding fans of sliced cheese and salami. At the center of the table stood the crystal starburst candleholders and violet-colored tapers I'd brought from Seattle for Zoya.

A zing of excitement hit me. Those were no ordinary tapers. They were World Peace candles. I had been waiting for the perfect moment to share their story with the Petrovy family. Now that moment was near.

After catching our breath, we all helped Zoya in the kitchen, where preparations for a feast were underway. Sergey pounded strips of beef on a cutting board and handed them to Zoya, who rolled each one with stuffing and baked them in the oven. Elina frosted a cake. Mike and I shuttled plates, cutlery, food, and condiments from the kitchen to the dining table. Vika opened a bottle of wine and cartons of juice. Maria stood beside the cupboard passing dishes, cutlery, and ingredients as needed to those trapped at their workstations without enough room to move. And Ivan paced in and out of the room carrying the baby over his shoulder.

As we performed this spontaneous ballet, the room pulsed with chatter and collisions of arms, tushes, and elbows followed by giggles and apologies. Ordinarily, in close quarters with that many people, I would have felt as though I were suffocating. Instead, I was basking in a delightful intimacy that illuminated the faint lines between chaos and symmetry, curiosity and fear, love and violence. The willingness to be fully present made all the difference.

When we were all seated at the table, Ivan uncapped the bottle of vodka. Vika struck a match to light the candles. There was no doubt in my mind, this was my moment. With my heart beginning to race, I took a deep breath.

"These candles were previously lit by a flame passed down from flames that were blessed by spiritual leaders on five continents," I explained. After a pause to allow Vika time to translate, I continued. "His Holiness the Dalai Lama, Archbishop Desmond Tutu, and Native American elders, among others, have blessed this flame."

Confusion passed over Vika's face. My words were met with silence. Suppressing my own confusion, I blew past those puzzling reactions and soldiered on.

"The original five flames were flown to Wales by military jets to be joined as one. That World Peace Flame is still burning in Wales and continues to spread around the world, from person to person, candle by candle."

Just as I was about to describe how I had received the flame at an interfaith church in Seattle, little Liya caught my attention with a deep gurgle. Drooling, the shiny-eyed baby bouncing on Sergey's knee smiled at me with a quirky, knowing grin.

Then my eyes opened wider. Maria, eager to move on to the booze and food, was drumming on the table with her long, painted fingernails. I realized there was not a glint of understanding in the room. Only blank stares, polite smiles, and silence. I concluded that Vika must have told her family, "I have no idea what Gail is saying, it's something about the candles."

My heart skipped a beat. Did they think I was making an excuse for why the purple tapers were already burned at the tips?

Years later, I wished my wiser self had been there to whisper in my ear, "Honey, this *is* a slice of world peace. You're living it, baby. Shut up or you'll miss it!"

But nooooo, I couldn't give it a rest. Gripped by an urge to tell them that sitting before us might actually be the first World Peace Flame to burn in Belarus, I took a breath. But before I could launch back into the story, Ivan, thinking my incomprehensible tale had ended, began filling shot glasses and proposed a toast.

"Za zdoroviy!" To health.

A voice inside my head protested, *No! Wait! I'm not finished!* Sensing my disappointment, Mike slipped an arm over my shoulder and squeezed, like Morse code: *It's okay, Gailey. I get you. Let it go now.*

While everyone else slugged down shots of vodka, I took a sip of wine and followed it with a dill pickle. Salads, smoked fish, potatoes, and stuffed beef swirled around the table. As conversation flew about the room in two languages, I puzzled over what had happened. Was it a simple case of a story completely lost in translation? Then it hit me: *Maybe they aren't familiar with the Dalai Lama or Desmond Tutu because, in Belarus, it's illegal to practice or promote any religion unauthorized by the government.*

Those thoughts led me down another rabbit hole. *Maybe the Petrovy family thinks I've brought contraband into their home!* With that, my stomach knotted. I pictured the KGB throwing me into a dungeon for smuggling evil candles into the country.

As my imagination spun out of control, Maria burst into another rock star performance, singing into her "microphone" fork, shaking her head and shoulders. Baby Liya gleefully babbled and swung her arms. Waves of chatter and laughter flooded the room. Realizing no one else was worried about candles or going to jail, I began to relax. Until Ivan proposed another toast.

"*Chai!*" he said, raising the bottle of vodka.

Everyone, including me, laughed at his reference to his mother's homemade vodka. But his humorous toast reminded me of the six-inch Irish crystal votive holder I'd given to Babushka along with an assortment of dried mushrooms, tea, and chocolate. The tea and food items were practical choices she could use. But Waterford crystal? *What was I thinking?*

I had assumed crystal was a good choice for Babushka because Zoya had sent gifts of Russian crystal to me when the girls had come to visit. And also because my mother and grandmother collected crystal vases, bowls, and goblets, as well as porcelain dishes. To hear the two of them talk, you might have thought they worshipped those collections more than they did their children, spouses, or God Almighty.

Like Babushka, my mother was hardworking and had grown up poor without the luxury of indoor plumbing. But Mom had access to a business school education after graduating from high school. As a young wife and mother, she had worn cinched-waist dresses, nylon stockings, garter belts, and high-heeled shoes to work. And if the cows were loose when she came home at five o'clock, she chased them into the barn still wearing those high heels.

Babushka was a force of a different nature. She still didn't have indoor plumbing. After a life of hardship, war, and physical labor, she was delighted not by *things* or appearances but by laughing, crying, singing, and drinking shots of home-distilled vodka with family and friends. Not an ounce of pretension lived under her skin.

Now, as I savored Zoya's *varenyky*—half-moons of hot dough stuffed with bits of smoked salmon from Seattle—a brilliant idea popped into my thoughts. *Next time I'll bring fresh king salmon! One for Zoya and Ivan and one for Babushka.* Then another voice in my head spoke up. *Are you out of your mind? You'd stink to high heaven and never clear customs. And think about the space those fish would take up in your suitcase. You brought too many bags as it is.*

Now I began stewing about my luggage. I was traveling with a boatload of nutritional supplements I hoped would protect my health, extra shoes, a book, a journal, and a heap of emergency food—energy bars, nuts, even cans of tuna fish. It hadn't seemed like too much before we'd left Seattle. But in Eastern Europe, our luggage had to be carried up and down dozens of stairs in buildings with no elevators and wheeled over rough ground. I had assumed they would be lightened when we unloaded the gifts we'd brought. But every time we presented a gift, we received one in return. So instead of getting lighter, our bags increased in weight. I cringed each time our male hosts insisted on carrying them for me.

Sitting at Zoya's table I now felt an urge to acknowledge that embarrassment. "I tried to bring small gifts," I began. "But our bags are still loaded to the gills!" I knew it had come out wrong the moment the words left my lips.

A hush fell over the table. I had just talked myself into another crevasse with no way out. Sounding like I was patting myself on the back for bringing so many gifts that it took two muscular men to carry them all, I was back where I had started. How could I have let this happen again?

"Gail?" Zoya's eyes smiled at me as she handed me her picture-perfect masterpiece of white mushroom caps poking through a twelve-inch round berm covered with a thick green coat of finely chopped dill and parsley.

Holding the heavy platter, I was grateful to be relieved of my thoughts. "*Chto eto?*"

"Mushroom meadow," Vika explained, a layered salad that included sliced boiled eggs, shredded cheese, smoked fish, and cabbage, all fused with mayonnaise and covered with herbs.

"*Krasivaya!*" I said, scooping a serving onto my plate. *Beautiful.*

Zoya watched as I raised a bite of the salad to my lips. To my delight, it tasted like a hybrid of tuna salad and coleslaw—tasty staples from my childhood. At long last, I came to my senses and stopped brooding. Turning to Zoya, I smiled.

"*Vkusno!*" I declared. *Tasty.* Zoya's face lit up, her eyes glowing with satisfaction.

In that moment, I understood that no explanation or apology was necessary. This family had a way of knowing my deepest intentions regardless of my faux pas—real or imagined. I took a long, slow breath, filling my lungs with the fragrance of care, attention, and love Zoya had poured into preparing this banquet for us in her little kitchen.

I turned my gaze to the people gathered around me. Sergey shifted the baby to her mother's lap and bent over his plate with gusto. Elina held a taste of potato to Liya's curlicue lips. Tilting her head, Maria looked at me with glittery green eyes and a mischievous smile that reminded me of her as a child. Vika pulled her chair away from the table, patted her flat belly, and groaned.

I was feeling what I'd felt at the Interfaith Community Sanctuary in the warm dazzling light of a hundred peace flames. The kiss of humankind. A sense of belonging. Knowing that each of us longs for the other, though our reach can be clumsy. I thought about the horrors of Khatyn, the senseless violence of war and genocide, and the one small bridge I had dreamed to life.

"To Zoya and Ivan!" I said, raising my glass of wine. "For sharing their daughters with Mike and me. And for keeping the doors open to their hearts and home."

Zoya's eyes met mine. "You made me a mama," I said, feeling gratitude in my bones. Even though I spoke in English, she understood.

"*Yi babushka!*" she added, lifting her chin toward Liya. *And grandmother.* Her blessing made me a proud mother and *babushka.*

Before we left the table, Ivan lifted his accordion to his lap. Filled with the elixir of belonging, my heart sang as sounds of the Old World danced around the room.

CHAPTER 31

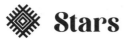 **Stars**

Belarus

As the end of our time in Belarus drew near, Zoya informed us that she, Elina, and the baby would travel with Mike and me back to Kyiv. There, he and I would transfer to a train to Vinnytsia, where Alex and Ella would be waiting. Though we assured her that wasn't necessary, she insisted.

"Mama say you not cross border or look for train in Kyiv without someone who speak Russian to help you," explained Maria. "Train station very big, Gail. Remember?"

On the day of our departure, Vlad drove us and the whole family to Minsk for our evening train. We arrived hours early to avoid any reason to rush or worry. After strolling in a city park, Mike and I came up with a brilliant idea, we thought. With extra time, why not take our Belarusian family to a restaurant as an expression of our gratitude for their hospitality? It didn't occur to us that this common practice in our culture might translate into a completely different experience in Belarus. Naturally, everyone was too polite to tell us our plan was a tad off-course.

The first obstacle was simply finding a restaurant. Our family wasn't familiar with any and Google was still so new that it wasn't a tool we used yet. So we walked up and down streets in search of a place to eat until Sergey remembered seeing a restaurant, Stars, located in the train station.

Seated at a long table, we were the only people in the restaurant besides the employees. The floor and bright purple walls were painted with silver stars. When Zoya opened a menu and saw the prices, she gasped. In response, I encouraged everyone to order whatever they wanted, never thinking that might make me sound like an imprudent American acting like a big shot.

When the waitress came for our orders, I realized nearly everyone at the table was still reticent. *Have we somehow offended them? Are they uncomfortable because they aren't able to reciprocate? Do they not realize how much they enhance our lives, that the gifts of our relationship flow both ways?* Searching for an answer, I turned to Maria and Vika.

"I don't understand. Why don't they want to eat?" Accustomed to eating in restaurants with us, the twins shrugged their shoulders nonchalantly. "Please, tell them Mike and I will feel bad if we eat more than they do."

My coaxing seemed to make a difference. Orders were placed, albeit reluctantly, but Mike and I wouldn't know what anyone had ordered until it appeared at the table. Taking much longer than expected, our orders dribbled out of the kitchen haphazardly. A side of cheesy potatoes with ham arrived first. Through the eyes of our Belarusian family, it must have looked like a puny serving for the price of a meal their whole family could eat at home. They laughed.

When everything had been delivered, Vlad had no food and Sergey had only a carafe of vodka he was sharing with Ivan. Mike and I couldn't decipher if they hadn't ordered anything or if the kitchen had screwed up. But we didn't have time to wait any longer, so we pleaded with Vlad and Sergey to share our food, and they complied politely.

I would have loved to know what the family thought about that madcap meal. By the time it ended we had to make a fast dash to collect our luggage from Vlad's van and hustle to the train. Elina and Zoya each carried one small duffel, though they and the baby would be staying with Babushka for the next ten days. Mike and I were down to five bags between us, still an embarrassment to me.

Standing outside our carriage before boarding, Maria draped her arm over my shoulder and Vika clasped my hand. I reached up with my other hand to hold Maria's. Ivan stood between Zoya and Mike, holding them both with his arms over their shoulders. Sergey mooned over Elina and the baby, missing them already.

Saying goodbye to the twins wasn't easy. "You'll always be my beautiful swimming fish girls," I said, kissing each of them with tears in my eyes. In the pregnant silence that followed was the unspoken question that had hung in the air each time they left Seattle. *Will we see each other face-to-face ever again?* Never knowing when politics or war might create a barrier between us was the awful price of making family with people in conflicting countries.

As we boarded the train, Sergey called out to Elina in English, "I love you!"

Mike and I stashed our bags and joined Zoya and Elina—with the baby in her arms—at the windows outside our side-by-side sleeping compartments, waving and throwing kisses. Using sign language—pointing to my eye, then my heart, then to the twins—I told the girls I loved them one last time before they faded out of sight.

A part of me stayed behind with them and a part of Belarus went with me. The place that had terrified me was now stitched into the universe of my interior, part of an unplanned spiritual journey that had begun, unbeknownst to me, when I was a child who longed for a world attuned to love instead of fear.

CHAPTER 32

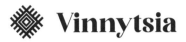 # Vinnytsia

Ukraine

As our train chugged out of Minsk, fears of being detained occupied only a teeny space in my subconscious. By the time we reached the Ukrainian border, I felt calm as a monk. Zoya sat with us for the inspection of our documents in the middle of the night, which ended quickly without an anxious moment.

When I awakened in the morning, we were approaching the chaos and confusion of the railway station in Kyiv, a mind-boggling hub with sixteen tracks and multiple buildings connected by bridges, all converging with the Metro subway system and a maze of suburban, regional, international, and airport trains. I was grateful for our chaperones. With baby Liya on Elina's hip and all of us weighed down with baggage, we climbed up and down stairs and threaded our way through swarms of people to reach the train to Vinnytsia.

After Mike and I kissed Elina and Liya goodbye, Zoya insisted on boarding the train with us to be certain we found two seats together in the crowded economy car; I suspect she was prepared to negotiate a seat swap for us if only singles were left. When the train was about to depart, she and I teared up. A long embrace conveyed what we knew in our hearts but couldn't speak. We were knitted together like the colorful wool "SOLMATES" I'd seen in stores: pairs of socks in complementary color palettes with rows of zigzags, lines, chevrons, and triangles that were harmoniously mismatched.

Zoya and Elina waved to us from the platform as our train pulled away. Taking a deep breath, I welcomed the pause, transition time between places and people. I needed the rest of anonymity, to enjoy hearing the music of conversations in a foreign language without the need to understand or engage. I could simply be.

While Mike read, I gazed out the window. Time seemed to stand still even as the train carried us one hundred and sixty miles southwest of Kyiv, across a panorama of fields, forests, and scattered communities. The rolling landscape and stuffy air lulled me into a languid state.

Ten minutes before we expected to arrive in Vinnytsia, Mike and I jockeyed our way toward the door with a crush of other passengers eager to exit the train in that city of 360,000 souls. The sweltering heat and a combination of garlic and body odors dizzied me. Still, I found myself smiling. After making the four-hour trip in the economy car with local people—instead of being isolated in first class—I felt like a new member of an insider's club.

Then, just before the train reached the station, it stopped. After an interlude, everyone looked around with questioning eyes. Still no movement or explanation.

Gradually, the crowd became more vocal and restless, but not alarmed, which kept me from imagining frightening scenarios. Some of the passengers had boarded the train in Moscow almost twenty-four hours earlier and had slept on boards attached to the walls. Those so-called beds looked to me like small surfboards that would throw you off every time the train rounded a curve or hit a rough spot. I guessed those were the passengers now at their wits' end, crying and hollering words I suspected were forbidden in polite conversation.

The conductor, offering no explanation for the delay, opened the door to let in a breeze. The circulation of air did make a little difference. But there was a tradeoff. Money-changers and elderly women selling sunflower seeds and strawberries stepped on board, trying to make a living. Stuck in the small area connecting two cars, those of us waiting to exit tried to move our bags out of their way. But there was no room to move. The *babushkas* and moneychangers ended up climbing over us and our belongings every time one of them stepped on or off or crossed from one carriage to the next. We passed bills, coins, and snacks back and forth between them and the customers they couldn't reach. Sweat ran down my face and back, and my head was spinning from dehydration. But there were no beverages available. After we had waited for forty-five minutes with no explanation, the train finally inched up to the platform.

"Welcome to Vinnytsia!" Alex beamed. Standing next to Ella, he held his arms out to greet us. I knew our safe arrival relieved him of worry. As our self-appointed leader, he felt responsible for our comfort and safety. Since the moment we'd arrived in Ukraine, he had stuck close by, never leaving us alone in public places. Maybe he worried we'd find ourselves impossibly lost or unable to communicate in a medical emergency, or that we might be easy prey for pickpockets and swindlers. I couldn't tell if he was projecting onto us the fears he had faced as an immigrant in the United States, or if Mike and I were surrounded by dangers we underestimated. Not for a moment did I feel unsafe.

Our arrival marked a milestone for Mike and me, completing our first solo travel in Ukraine, and for Alex and Ella, completing a circle connecting their life in the United States with their roots. Soon they would introduce us to their Ukrainian friends and family.

"I have good news!" Alex announced. "We have room for you at Hotel Podillia. We will take you there now to rest for a couple hours before we show you the city."

Hallelujah! I needed to reset my internal circuit breakers with a bottle of cold water and a long shower.

"Also, bad news," added Alex. "Water in hotel not working."

"Don't worry," said Ella. "Will be fixed by ten o'clock this evening."

I wasn't so sure. A moment of paranoia hit me. *What if the water problem can't be fixed? What if the whole city winds up without drinking water? We'll be caught in a bottled water war!* Those thoughts seemed extreme even to me.

"At least we can have a nap and regroup," I said cheerfully, pushing those ridiculous thoughts out of my consciousness.

The Podillia couldn't have been more to my liking. Standing stones carved with faces and animals were scattered like totems on the grounds of the hotel, a low-rise building that appeared a bit dated but well-maintained. A friendly desk clerk apologized for the plumbing situation, assured us it would be fixed soon, and handed us our room key and tickets for breakfast the next morning.

"Is bottled water available here?" I inquired.

"Yes. Machine near elevator, just over there," he said, pointing to the other side of the lobby. Mike and I exchanged smiles. Cold water in a vending machine *and* an elevator!

A soft Turkish-style rug carpeted the floor of the elevator, a modern luxury we hadn't expected. Our homey fifth-floor quarters felt more like a European apartment than a hotel room. Soft white curtains and linens covered the windows and twin beds. A lovely Euro-style combination window-door opened to a balcony. Surrounded by a perfect mix of quaint and modern touches, I felt at home.

"Gailey, come see this view!" said Mike, stepping outside.

A sea of green trees, dotted with rooftops, stretched all the way over a high plateau in the distance. Standing behind Mike with my arms wrapped around him, I took several long, slow, deep breaths and began to unwind. After a dreamy nap on the bed beside the open door, I felt renewed when our friends came back for us, ready for the change of plans I'd come to expect on this trip.

"New plan!" announced Alex. He and Ella had learned early in life that adapting to unexpected change was critical to their survival in Ukraine. That lesson had become second nature to them.

"Tamara wants us to go to the cemetery with her." Tamara was Alex's only sibling, his grief-stricken older sister who lived alone. Years earlier, her husband had died. Now she was also grieving the recent death of her son, an only child.

"We take food and flowers to put on graves. Special custom in Ukraine," Ella explained.

"It sounds like a very intimate ritual, and I don't want to intrude. Maybe it's better if Mike and I wait here," I suggested.

"No, not intrude," responded Ella. "Tamara ask us to bring you. She understands you are family." I felt deeply honored.

On the way to Tamara's apartment, Alex explained that his brother-in-law and nephew had both died of heart attacks, years apart.

"Did they have a genetic heart condition?" I asked.

"We don't know. Maybe genetics. Maybe radiation," Alex speculated. "They both worked with television and radio antennas, exposing them to radiation. When Chernobyl explode, they get even more exposure."

Tall and dignified, Tamara wore a headscarf over her shoulder-length, chestnut-brown hair. Her small apartment was still and dark but not bleak. It felt as if a river of grace had spilled into the room from her broken heart, and the force of that river kept her alive. After she embraced Mike and me, she handed Ella and me each a headscarf.

"We wear these to the cemetery," said Ella, "to show respect." We placed them on our heads and tied them under our chins, as Tamara had done.

The graveyard, on the outskirts of town, reminded me of a large overgrown garden divided into dozens of small plots. Tamara led us down a dirt path past row after row of plots, each one outlined with concrete curbs and marked with tombstones or crosses fashioned from painted metal pipes. Despite her burden of grief and tears, she carried herself with the elegance of a dancer, her spine straight, her movements fluid, intentional, and light.

We turned between two rows and walked down a lane overgrown with weeds and wildflowers until we reached the side-by-side graves of Tamara's spouse and son. Weeping, she seated herself on the ground, opened the bag she'd carried with her, and removed its contents. Gardening gloves. Tools. A bottle of water to pour on the plants.

As Tamara dug up weeds from her husband's grave with an old, clawed tool, her tears fell to the ground and birds sang in a nearby forest. Ella created an altar of food and juice on the baked earth covering her nephew's plot. It was too soon after his death, less than a year, to plant flowers or place a stone on his grave, Ella said.

When Tamara finished weeding and watering, she stood, and Ella handed each of us two long-stemmed roses to place on the graves. In keeping with their funeral traditions, she made sure that an even number of flowers wound up on each one. Then we all sat on the ground. Alex, Ella, and Tamara cried together and talked in their native tongue. Though I couldn't participate in sharing memories or expressing words of comfort, I felt connected and engaged by bearing witness to Tamara's pain and loss. I knew that in some cultures, grief could not be healed until it was witnessed, and the deceased could only reach their ancestors in the afterlife on a river of tears.

After a long, quiet pause, Tamara invited us to eat the bite-sized confections on the altar. Ella handed each of us a paper cup and filled it with juice. Alex made a somber toast to one of life's most precious and most painful moments.

Tamara wailed as we returned to the car, leaning into me as though I were a sister. I wrapped my arm over her shoulder and held her close, helping to carry her grief for a short while.

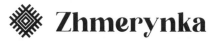 Zhmerynka

Ukraine

"All Jewish people lived on this street," said Ella, her tone somber and sad. We were walking down the long, sloping street in Zhmerynka where my Jewish friend and Alex had lived with their daughter before moving to America. "Now, all gone," added Ella as we walked past shopkeepers sweeping the doorways of their small convenience stores.

Farther downhill, she stopped in front of a crumbling building with a door propped open. "This was Jewish synagogue," she said. Signs of neglect and battered doors left me with the impression that no one had stepped inside in years. But I couldn't be sure.

"Is it still used?" I asked. A light breeze carried the gleeful shrieks of children playing in the street.

"Some people still live in this building. When Communists came into power, they banned religion and make synagogue into apartments," explained Ella.

That ban had been put in place long before Ella's birth. She remembered her grandmother going to someone else's house to pray in secrecy. Before Communist rule, Zhmerynka had once been the home of seven synagogues and three Jewish schools.

After the collapse of the Soviet Union, when Jews were permitted to leave the country, "All the Jewish people go to Israel, US, and Germany," said Ella. "All over. Like us."

"Did they leave because of how the Jews were treated during the pogroms and the Holocaust?" It made sense to me that they would want to leave the land where Jews had suffered collective trauma for centuries.

"No, that was a different generation," she said dispassionately. "We left because the economic situation was not good. We went to find better opportunities."

Ella's emotional detachment perplexed me. Her father, who had moved to the United States a couple of years ahead of her, had asked that, while we were in Ukraine, we locate the field where his aunt and cousin had been shot dead and buried in a mass grave with other Jews. We were planning to visit the site that very day. Trying to understand how Ella carried that history, and knowing she always welcomed my questions, I pressed further.

"But Ella, only fifty years had passed between the end of the Holocaust and your move to Seattle. Didn't you live with the weight of that history or feel the presence of ghosts from the past when you lived in Zhmerynka?"

"No, not," she said with certainty.

I flashed back to the dissonance I felt when Zoya had talked about Chernobyl as if it were ancient history with no ongoing consequences to their well-being. Now, I was experiencing a moment of déjà vu with Ella.

It didn't dawn on me until much later that Ella and Zoya might both have been numb to the impact of the tragedies their families had experienced. My training as a mental health counselor had taught me that emotional detachment was a hallmark of trauma survivors and people who inherit a legacy of unresolved trauma from their ancestors—especially those with no safe place to talk about the horrors. Ella had been unable to openly acknowledge or discuss the targeting of Jews while living in the Soviet Union, and Zoya still couldn't publicly question the information provided by the government regarding the effects of radiation exposure. Detachment could have been protecting them from anguish, like a Band-Aid that shouldn't be ripped off until it's safe. Maybe those traumas were still too close, too raw, not yet safe for Ella or Zoya to reckon with. As I mulled over the terrible realities my dear friends carried with them, a quote by novelist Rachel Kadish came to mind: "Truth telling is a luxury for those whose lives aren't at risk."

I was beginning to melt in the sun when we caught up with Mike and Alex, standing in front of an old building with concrete siding. I thought it was a dilapidated warehouse with no windows and two big blue doors. Brick was exposed in places where the siding had broken off.

"Go inside," said Alex, lifting his chin toward the building. "Special treat just for you, Ella." Ella's face brightened and we headed for the door.

"This is the gymnasium in my old school," she said. "My daughter went to school here too. My mother was a teacher here."

A different world awaited us inside the doors. Folk music filled the air, and a group of teenage girls dressed in traditional Ukrainian attire were dancing onstage in front of an audience. With bright smiles, red lipstick, and matching red ribbons holding back their hair, the dancers glowed with a mesmerizing radiance. Their white peasant-style *vyshyvanky*—blouses adorned with embroidered Ukrainian motifs—were tucked into pomegranate-red skirts that fell to their knees in lovely drapes and swirled like silk. Bold red

flowers were stitched on the sleeves of their blouses, a deli-
cate geometric pattern graced their necklines, and their skirts
were embroidered with colorful symbols that reminded me
of hieroglyphics.

Ella and I sat close to the front. Captivated by the charming dancers, and the music, colors, and choreography, I didn't
realize, until the director stopped the music to make changes
in the routine, this was a dress rehearsal for an upcoming
performance.

Dressed for a special occasion, most of the spectators
were women. Some of them smiled and waved to Ella. After
the rehearsal, they greeted her and peppered her with questions. Unable to participate in those conversations, I slipped
outdoors to sit on the steps in the shade.

While I waited outside, people walked by staring at me.
I smiled, assuming they were surprised to see a foreigner
in town. When Alex came and sat next to me, I assumed
he'd come to keep me company. Years later I would learn
that both of my assumptions were wrong. The townspeople
were staring at me because, in that part of the world, people
believed that sitting on the steps or the ground (unless the
ground was covered by a cloth) could make you ill. Alex
had joined me to make me more comfortable while being
scrutinized for my improper and risky behavior.

We continued walking when Ella rejoined us. "Did you
talk with any of your Jewish friends?" I asked.

"No Jewish people here. All gone." Though she had told
me that earlier, I hadn't taken it literally.

"Many people were happy to see you," I remarked.

"Yes, they are very curious," she said. "They ask me
about our life in the US, and they ask why you would want
to come here. They don't understand."

"What did you tell them?"

"I say it is interesting for you, a different experience, and I tell about the family you came to visit. They surprised you friends for many years," she said.

I wondered if my friendship with Ella puzzled them too. In Denmark, where Mike and I had once stayed in a villa owned by Jews, the local non-Jewish people we met asked why we didn't choose a different hotel. Taken aback by this attitude, which we encountered several times, we told them, "We are Americans. We don't have any problems with staying in a Jewish hotel." I knew that anti-Semitism existed in the United States, but it was less obvious at that time than racism. Except in Denmark, I had never, to my knowledge, encountered anti-Semitism firsthand. In my culture, it was often hidden in plain sight.

At the foot of the street, we stood in front of Alex and Ella's former home, a one-bedroom, one-story whitewashed house they sold before leaving the country. It had the same tin roof and outhouse my friends remembered. In front of the property stood the same fence, a tall barrier pieced together with wood and pipes painted aqua green. The only sign of change or progress Alex noted was a satellite dish attached to the house. This represented a huge step forward, one that connected the current residents to global news that wasn't accessible during the Soviet era.

A blonde woman wearing a colorful sundress came out to see who was standing at her gate. She greeted us like old friends, and Ella introduced herself and her entourage. The woman said she now lived in the house with her husband and two daughters and invited us in for tea. At first Ella declined, not wanting to impose, but when the woman insisted, we gladly followed her inside.

Tidy, sparsely furnished, and showing signs of age but

not neglect, it felt like a happy home where dreams were born. First, Alex and Ella's dream to live in the United States, followed by the teenage girl now sitting with a computer on her lap, studying for a college entrance exam—in a home that still had no indoor toilet, tub, or shower. Though I had grown accustomed to the confluence of New World and Old World on this trip, I felt jarred and surprised every time it confronted me like that.

The lines between joy and sorrow, contemporary and antiquated, barely existed in this culture. Ukraine was a coin with creativity and hope on one side, tragedy and loss on the other. It flipped constantly. Alex and Ella had adapted to crossing those lines regularly and abruptly, but it felt like whiplash to me.

After we paid homage to Ella and Alex's former home with tea and conversation, we walked back up the street. Wrung out from the heat, we paused in the town square at the top before heading out on our mission for Ella's father. A new, red brick Orthodox Christian church crowned with metallic gold domes dominated that prominent place, once a Mecca for Jews. The full meaning and symbolism of that new jewel eluded me in that moment. I viewed it as a sign of prosperity growing in a new democracy. Alex and Ella posed in the square with Mike and me for a photo, set against the backdrop of the domes ablaze with sunlight. Only later would I see the terrible incongruity of that scene, sandwiched between the street once populated with Jews and our next stop—the place where Ella's relatives were murdered just outside of town.

There was no sign marking the entrance to the New Jewish Cemetery of Brailov. We drove past the turnoff several times before spotting the two-track road and following it into a field. Almost hidden by trees and undergrowth, a handful of leaning tombstones dotted one end of the cemetery. The recently installed tomb-like monument occupied the other end. Standing about six feet high and more than fifty feet long, it seemed out of place in the middle of the field, without even a fence to contain all that it concealed.

Alex parked the car in a clearing and we walked in silence to the memorial. It was the color of dark, angry storm clouds. I put my hand on its rough surface, as though I needed to make sure it was real. Attached to the front side were plaques engraved with the names of the victims. Unable to read Cyrillic, Mike and I were of no help in the search for the names of Ella's kin.

As I stood in silence, a flashback of my recent trip to Khatyn, in Belarus, reminded me that, once again, I was standing in a killing field on a paradoxically beautiful day. This was not what I had expected to be doing on this trip. But we were not tourists on vacation. We hadn't come to visit beaches, hike trails, or sample foods in all the restaurants. I was not there to simply observe. I had come prepared to immerse myself in the culture of loved ones whose lives had been shaped so differently than mine. I was there learning to grow into the skin of a global citizen.

This couldn't happen in the US, I kept thinking. But it *had* happened in the United States, multiple times. The attempted genocide of Indigenous Americans. The building of our nation on a foundation of enslaved Black people. Institutionalized racism. Ongoing police brutality and murder of people of color. Anti-Semitism on the rise.

Was I numb to the collective trauma of violence in my own country? Was my psyche trying to protect *me* with a dose of denial? Did the persistence of injustice keep us all anesthetized? I hadn't anticipated how significantly this trip would expand my vision of my own culture—a necessary part of becoming a global citizen.

When Alex and Ella located the names of her family members, the discovery evoked no tears or visible signs of emotion, only a simple acknowledgment. The moment seemed deserving of something more, but I had no frame of reference, no precedent to follow. It was Mike who broke the silence.

"Millions of people killed like this." He shook his head in disbelief.

"This is just what happened," remarked Ella, with a shrug of resignation.

"How did your father and the rest of his family survive?" I asked her.

"They went to Uzbekistan until the war ended." She didn't say how they knew when to leave, how they traveled or had the means to do so.

Though I didn't know it yet, I was learning how other cultures face and grieve an unbearable past in order to heal. The monument at Brailov served as an official acknowledgment of the state's responsibility for that massacre. The United States still hadn't taken that step; many of our monuments and institutions still glorified those who enslaved and fought to maintain slavery, and colonizers responsible for slaughtering Native Americans.

Only years later would I learn that the mass grave at Brailov was just one of more than sixty blanketing the bucolic countryside surrounding Vinnytsia. Thousands upon thousands of victims of Soviet secret police and Nazi massacres lay under that ground. No wonder I had experienced a wave of paranoia in Vinnytsia when I first arrived on the train!

That day, we left the Brailov cemetery in a somber mood that would soon shift again when we reached the home of Ella's friend Irina. Irina served us a special treat, new potatoes fresh from her garden. When I tasted the boiled potatoes, drizzled with butter, salt, and dill, my taste buds brought me back to the joys of being alive. While I savored those flavors, Irina's eight-year-old granddaughter and her two friends eyed me with big smiles and missing teeth from their seats across the table. Their curiosity reminded me of myself as a young girl drawn to the foreigners who weeded our fields. But this trio of giggling girls was braver than me. After we finished eating, instead of keeping their distance, as I had done, they invited me to join them in a game.

It was the old, familiar game of building a tower by taking turns placing our hands on top of each other's, then each of us pulling a hand out when it reached the bottom, and placing it on top, picking up speed until all our hands were slapping each other's, our arms were all tangled, and we were overcome with laughter. Then we started over.

Their little pancake hands stacked together with my adult ones connected us to the magic of touch and humor and cut straight through the walls of separation between those three young bridge builders and me without any shared language except laughter. I tried to picture those little Ukrainian girls in the future, and I hoped their curiosity and openness would survive whatever life brought to their doorsteps.

The next day, while Alex and Ella remained for a longer visit in Vinnytsia, Mike and I returned to Kyiv for our flight back to Seattle. Completing the circle, Zoya met us at the airport to see us off with one last embrace, one last kiss.

Going home, I was not the same person I'd been when I arrived. My picture of motherhood—and myself—had been transformed when Zoya recognized me as the honorary mother and *babushka* of her daughters and grandchild. The history I'd felt and witnessed in Belarus and Ukraine had given me a perspective of the world almost impossible to acquire growing up in the United States, a country still in its infancy and sitting at the top of the world's power structure. I'd made peace with infertility and with a family of former Soviets still living in the shadow of the Iron Curtain.

Part Seven:
2014

CHAPTER 34

❖ Love and War

In 2014, just emerging from a vortex of grief and loss, Mike and I were making plans to finally reunite with the twins, in Belarus. Since our first trip to their country, Mike had suffered a heart attack and, over a five-year period, all four of our parents had died.

To my great disappointment, due to the upheaval in our lives, we had been unable to attend Vika's wedding. Now she had a son, Nikita, who was almost three years old.

I longed to meet Fedor, the young man who had captured Vika's heart. I ached to hold Vika's child and Elina's new baby boy, Ivan, to smell the sweetness of their soft skin, and to search the depths of their eyes for glimmers of wisdom they might one day share with the world.

But in April 2014, Russia invaded Ukraine and seized the Crimean Peninsula. The United States condemned the annexation and imposed sanctions on Russia. A violent campaign to secede parts of eastern Ukraine followed. Lines of war were drawn with Russia and Belarus on one side, Ukraine and the United States on the other. Concerned that we could be targets for anti-Western hostility in Belarus, or worse, caught in a war zone, Mike and I put our travel plan on hold. We were still waiting to see what developed before canceling and disappointing the twins, when Maria called from Minsk.

Dim lighting and a fuzzy Skype connection painted her on my screen in shades of gray and black. Her eyes popped out through dark circles of fatigue and eyeliner.

"Mama need passport numbers for you. She start paperwork for you to come to us this summer." Her tone sounded urgent.

A lump lodged in my throat. Was she aware of the violence escalating in Ukraine? We sometimes heard what was going on in Belarus and its neighboring countries before it was announced in Belarus.

Trying to summon the courage to tell her our plans were now on hold, and why, I glanced outside my windows. Spring rain drizzled down the glass and dark clouds hovered over the Olympic Mountains. My stomach churned with resentment. *Why do we even have to have this conversation?* I felt caught in a fifty-year time warp, reliving the Cold War. My longing to see the girls again ran deep and I would do almost anything to avoid disappointing them.

Now, I drew my gaze back to the screen where twenty-five-year-old Maria sat on her bed, her long legs stretched out in front of her on a flowered spread. She looked terribly young and alone against the bare walls of her small room.

I took a breath. "Maria, I hope we can come this summer," I said, choosing my words carefully. "We have to wait and see what happens with Russia and Ukraine." Her face tightened. Her lips puckered.

"I *know*, Gail." She sounded like a teenager responding to a parent's constant warnings to be wary of strangers. She didn't want to hear it. Her strategy for coping with danger was to avoid seeing it as long as possible. "Is bad now. Maybe soon is better." She folded her legs up and peered at me with feral eyes. I had pierced her protective barrier.

"Are you worried?"

"Yes. Everybody worried," she said, as though confessing a weakness. She had been the sassy, fearless twin who threw caution to the wind as a child. Scrambling to the top of a rock-climbing wall, then leaning back into a fall, trusting her harness to hold as she belayed her way down. Running to the end of a high diving board and jumping into the water without hesitation. Calling to me from the top of a Ferris wheel, "Look, Gail! I standing!" She was also the one who'd often come to my room in the night to whisper in my ear, "Gail, I scared." Pulling back the covers, I'd let her slip in next to me where I could feel her heartbeat as she slept in my arms until she reverted to her invincible self in the morning.

Now, I wanted to snuggle up to her and tell her that all would be well in the morning. But I couldn't. By morning she could wake up to army tanks thundering through the streets, aimed for Ukraine.

"What are you most worried about?" I asked Maria, wishing I could slip my arm over her shoulder. Though I couldn't comfort her in person, I could at least employ my therapist skills and encourage her to talk about her fears.

"Maybe we can't go to Ukraine. Papa worried not see Babushka. She old, Gail, not feel good."

A sharp breath stabbed my chest. I pictured the starry night we spent at Babushka's, where four generations of her family had gathered around a table with Mike and me. I gazed at Maria through the screen. She sighed, then closed her eyes and tipped her head back against the wall.

"What else are you worried about?" I asked.

After a long pause, she opened her eyes. They were filled with sorrow. "People worried sons and brothers and uncles have to fight, maybe," she said, her voice hardly more than a whisper now. My mind flashed back to an image of the grieving women in black on the Isle of Tears in Minsk.

A weight landed in my stomach. My attempts to be objective vanished. This was personal, and I, too, felt scared. The possibility that Elina's and Vika's husbands would be forced to fight against their own families sickened me. I thought about the night in Ukraine, at Babushka's, when the twins' cousins had shared laughter, tears, and song with us. The girls always referred to them as their *brots. Brothers.* It was despicable that, on a whim, a government could tear out stitches of connection between brothers and sisters, aunts, uncles, and cousins by framing them as enemies. I prayed this tight-knit family wouldn't be made to face each other at gunpoint.

"Do you think Fedor and Sergey might be called for military duty?" Trying to conceal my own fears, I kept my voice even and steady.

"I don't know, Gail. Maybe you know more than we do. We hear only little."

I shuddered. The innocence of childhood no longer shielded Maria. At the same time, I felt the relief of knowing she understood, to some extent, how censorship in Belarus might impact her. I wished that I could protect her and her family from the complex and dangerous political conflict seeping into her life. Yet I couldn't even find words to comfort her. The threat of destruction that had riddled my childhood with fear brought the twins and me together through the portal of a nuclear disaster. Now, two generations later, it was poised to keep us apart. My heart ached. After we said goodbye, my heart sank as Maria's image faded from the screen.

Weeks flew by and the political situation worsened. Mike and I became increasingly worried. Knowing we needed to cancel our trip, we Skyped with the twins to discuss a new plan.

"Why don't you come to Seattle for a month," Mike proposed.

"Nikita and Liya too," I added.

Vika's and Maria's eyes grew wide. They turned to each other, then back to us.

"Yes, we come!" Vika said.

It had been thirteen years since their last trip to the United States, when they were twelve years old. Racing against time, they immediately embarked on the long, complicated process of obtaining US visas.

The embassy in Belarus could no longer issue visas. Instead, the girls applied at the embassy in Ukraine. The process would require two trips to Kyiv: One to deliver their completed applications and fees in person. A second trip for an in-person interview after the applications were processed, which also required Liya's parents and Nikita's father to be present to guarantee the travelers weren't planning to defect.

"If one mistake make on document, they say no, we lose all money and have to start over," Maria wailed. At my urging, she enlisted the help of her friend Yulia.

With Yulia's help, the applications were completed. Maria was delegated to make the first trip to Kyiv alone to deliver the finished paperwork and fees. Sleeping on a hard bench on the overnight train, she held the bag containing the money and documents tight to her chest. Though she had traveled to Ukraine many times with no trouble, this time when she reached the border, the guards treated Maria as a potential threat. They questioned her reasons for multiple trips into the country. Ukraine was her motherland, she explained, she traveled there often to visit her grandmother, cousins, aunts, and uncles—all Ukrainians, like her. That seemed to have meant little to the guards, but they allowed her to enter.

Shaken by the experience, Maria called to tell us what had happened. "I tell them I come for US visa, and next time I go back for interview. They say 'Maybe no next time.' I very scared."

For the second trip, they drove to Kyiv and there were no problems crossing the border. Maria emailed us the news from the embassy.

"They say yes! We go to office for documents in three days."

"I'm doing the happy dance!" I responded.

"We too!"

Allowing extra time for unexpected delays, Mike made their reservations on a flight departing from Kyiv in five days. But when the girls returned to the office to claim their visas, they learned the computer system had crashed. There were no visas. No one could say when the problem would be resolved. They were stuck waiting in Ukraine.

"People crying and screaming in visa office," Maria told us on Skype.

"Every day they say, 'Maybe tomorrow,'" Vika moaned.

The day of their flight came and went. The war intensified while they continued to wait. Ukrainian men between the ages of eighteen and sixty were prohibited from crossing the border into Belarus. Tanks overtook more villages. Then, a Malaysian commercial airliner carrying 295 passengers was shot down over eastern Ukraine by a surface-to-air missile. None of the passengers or crew survived. That tragedy sparked yet another change of plans.

"We no fly from Ukraine," said Maria. She sounded frightened. "Papa say after we get visa we go back to Belarus, fly from Minsk."

Every day of waiting meant one less day in Seattle because their return date couldn't be extended. Vika and Maria needed to resume working. Liya had to be back for school. And Nikita would lose his place in day care if he missed the first day.

Finally, the visas were issued. While our travelers headed back to Belarus, Mike, knowing it would be difficult to book four seats on international flights on short notice, especially out of Minsk, called the airline and explained the situation to a Delta reservation agent. Hearing we were former Children of Chernobyl volunteers, she went to bat for our Belarusian children and grandchildren, cobbled together an itinerary that would put them in the sky the following morning, and waived the fees normally charged for changing flights. We were ecstatic.

"You have to change planes in Vienna *and* in Amsterdam," Mike explained to Maria and Vika on Skype. Their only experience with air travel had been their trips to Seattle with Children of Chernobyl chaperones. This would be their first flight on their own, with two small children under their wings. But Mike and I never doubted their bravery or skills.

Anxious smiles and a hint of excitement registered on their faces. They'd never dreamed they'd step foot in Austria or Netherlands, even if it was only to make a transfer at the airport.

"You'll be okay. People will help you," Mike assured them. "You need to be at the airport in Minsk really early, no later than four thirty tomorrow morning."

"Don't worry, Mike. We go to airport at *three*," declared Maria.

With the arrangements in place, a manic impulse took hold of me. Like a woman about to go into labor, I began writing grocery lists, plumping pillows, and feathering my nest. Liya, now seven, had been an infant when we last saw her. I could hardly believe she, Vika's son Nikita, and the twins would soon walk through my door.

Feeling as though I were walking on clouds, I dashed outside to water the garden and cut flowers. Snipping sky-blue hydrangeas, I recalled the dinner when Zoya had recognized me as a mother and *babushka*. My interior landscape was changed by that gift, by feeling truly seen.

I wasn't a traditional mother or grandmother, but my unconventional making of family was real. The foursome now headed my way were as close to children and grandchildren as I would ever have. Though I had experienced only a handful of the important events in their lives, I hoped those shared experiences would be as meaningful and life-changing for them as they were for me. I was thrilled to have a new generation crossing our bridge, especially given that tensions between the United States and Russia were now at an all-time high since the ending of the Cold War. History was repeating itself.

While I arranged the hydrangeas in pretty glass vases handed down by my mother, my mind was spinning with questions. *Can we make up for lost time? Will Nikita need diapers? Will my relationship with Vika and Maria resemble the kind of relationship I had hoped to have as a mother with grown daughters?*

I glanced at the clock. *The girls are boarding their flight about now.* Just then, my cell phone pinged with an email notification. *They're letting me know they've boarded!* I grabbed the phone and opened the message.

"We at airport. They say we no board plane, maybe we arrested if we board plane. We need EU visa to go to Vienna."

My heart sank. *Damn!* The agent had said that because they wouldn't be leaving the airport in Vienna, they wouldn't need a transit visa. While that flight left the ground without them, I typed a response. "Don't worry. We will contact the airline and get back to you."

Looking back, I realize that message might have sounded as if we possessed the powers of a magic wand or a high-ranking official to pull strings. The girls may even have believed that. But our power had sprung from the privileges of US citizens with access to corporate jobs that paid well and offered perks. Mike had accrued a zillion air miles from business travel and was determined to use them to the girls' advantage.

Fueled with adrenaline, Mike and I went to work using every device at our disposal to reach a "special issues" airline agent. On the verge of panic, I waited on hold on my cell phone and on a landline while Mike, his face tight with determination, waited on his cell phone and simultaneously scanned flight information on two computer screens. Finally, he got through and explained the new situation. Thirty minutes later, four tickets were emailed to our weary travelers, for a flight leaving the next morning.

"Go home and get some sleep," Mike emailed.

"No Mike. We sleep in car at airport."

I pictured a small car in the airport parking lot with the twins, Elina, Sergey, and the two children all packed inside trying to sleep.

"They're going to be wiped out when they get here," I remarked.

"So are we!" Mike answered. Teal blue stars twinkled in his eyes. Crow's-feet radiated like beams of starlight at his temples. "I'm ready for a piña colada. Are you?" There in those blue pools of light I once again saw a wise and ancient soul, my North Star, this time masquerading as a bartender.

"Sure!" I said without hesitation, though I wasn't much of a drinker. "Maybe I'll have two!"

Indeed, I did have two drinks that evening in place of dinner—a first for me. Also out of character, I took my cell phone to bed with me in case there were any further hurdles.

Sure enough, just as Mike and I were drifting off to sleep, a *ping* sounded from my phone. We both sat up as I grabbed my Samsung in the dark. Holding my breath, I opened a new email from Maria.

"We sit on plane."

Mike and I both teared up. Our three-week three-ring circus was about to begin. We didn't yet know what that summer had in store for us: Fourteen dental appointments between our four guests, including oral surgery for Nikita. A betrayal that would whip up a squall. Little rest, plenty of drama, and enough joy to float an American *babushka* to the moon and back.

CHAPTER 35

❖ A New Constellation

S tationed at the top of the escalator, I scanned the stream of passengers coming up the moving stairs from customs to baggage claim. Security policies put in place after the 9/11 terrorist attacks prevented us from being able to see international passengers in the customs queues, as we could when the Children of Chernobyl groups arrived.

The waiting seemed endless. Many passengers from the twins' flight had already cleared customs, and still there was no sight of them.

"What if there's a problem?" I asked Mike. "We have no way of knowing." I felt a knot of anxiety tightening in my chest.

"Give it time," he said. Tension in his face told me he was worried too.

Just as the waiting became almost unbearable and my anxiety was morphing to panic, I saw a little light-haired fellow standing at the bottom of the stairs. A pair of eyeglasses sat cockeyed on his face. My heart began to race.

"Is that Nikita?" A young girl with braided hair walked up to the toddler and grabbed his hand.

"Yup! And Liya!"

"I see Maria and Vika right behind them!"

Tears sprung to my eyes and I couldn't stand still. My anxiety flew away and disappeared as I bounced and clapped. After helping the younger children step onto the escalator, the twins looked up and spotted Mike and me. The four of us broke into uncontainable smiles of joy and relief. It had been a long and challenging trip for our Belarusian family. Vika and Maria were not accustomed to negotiating major airports, stepping onto escalators with children who had probably never seen one before, and communicating with government officials in English. Not to mention fleeing a country under invasion, missing flights, and sleeping in the car.

The years of separation vanished like invisible ink when the twins stepped off the escalator and into our arms. After long-awaited hugs, we presented the girls with roses before kneeling to welcome the children with stuffed animals: a pink-nosed bunny for Liya and a bear for Nikita. Seven-year-old Liya threw her arms around my neck and held on tight, ready to embrace the unfamiliar with the same readiness I had seen in her the first time I held her in my arms, in Belarus, when she was just six months old. Nikita stared at us, probably wondering why we spoke only one word that made any sense to him: *privet*. Hi. I fell madly in love with him and Liya, right there in the airport.

We collected their small bags and hurried home to settle in. After the traditional gifting ritual, it was time for a meal.

"You must be starving," I said.

"Yes, we hungry," admitted Maria. "I make Russian pizza for you and the children, okay, Gail?"

"You don't need to cook. I have food already prepared. It just needs to be warmed up."

"You make tomorrow, Gail," Vika suggested. "The children like this food."

"Okay. Whatever you think is best." My role had shifted.

Now I was a grandmother and the twins were parenting. It was a change I welcomed.

"I'll take the kids outdoors," offered Mike. "I borrowed a police car for toddlers from a neighbor. I think Nikita is going to like it."

Vika scooped Nikita up into her arms, danced around the room with him, then devoured him with kisses while he squealed with delight. He was a boy who required constant engagement, and she happily complied. "You want to go outside with Mike?" she asked him in Russian. "He has a police car for you to drive!"

"*Da!*" Nikita responded. Without a moment of hesitation, he and Liya followed Mike out the door while the twins took over the newly remodeled kitchen.

Maria went to work, making a paste of flour and mayonnaise, spreading it across the bottom of a skillet, and heating it on the black glass-top stove that had replaced the old model I had treasured. Vika placed another skillet on the stovetop, sliced a zucchini fresh from my garden, and dropped the discs into hot sizzling oil after they were coated with beaten egg and dredged with flour. Cupboard doors hung open and the wood floor was dusted with flour. With the twins back in my orbit, my universe buzzed with excitement, creativity, and love.

"I put more mayonnaise, then ketchup on top. Pizza finish when everything hot!" Maria announced.

"No cheese?"

"No, only ketchup and mayonnaise. Is very good! I make this when I tired from work."

I wanted to suggest adding other ingredients from my refrigerator, but I resisted. This was a moment to experience a taste of the girls' normal life in Belarus and share their pride in their culinary skills.

"We buy Heinz ketchup to take to Zalessie?" Vika asked.

"Of course!" We always bought giant Costco-sized bottles of ketchup—one of the girls' favorite "sauces"—for them to take home.

Nikita's happy squeals, Mike's cheers, and the sounds of plastic tires rolling over concrete floated in through the open windows. As I stood basking in the twins' presence, I remembered the first dinner they made for us in our kitchen, when they were eight years old. Vika, wearing sunglasses to keep her eyes from watering as she diced onions, had perched on a stack of phone books to reach the cutting board. Maria had paced nervously, keeping her eye on pots of eggs, potatoes, and peas nearly boiling over on the old chrome-trimmed stove.

Now they were grown women, but the spark of life they ignited in me remained unchanged. I still felt as though I belonged to them and they belonged to me. I still wanted to give them the stars and the moon.

Maria squirted ketchup over the pizza. Vika stacked the fried zucchini slices on a plate, frosted the crisp, golden towers with mayonnaise, and set them on the table.

Mike strolled in from playing outdoors with the kids. "What can I do to help?"

"Pour drinks?" I suggested.

"Ok. Let's see," he said, opening the refrigerator, "we have milk, juice, or water."

Vika raised her eyebrows and smiled coyly. "Mike, maybe you make piña coladas?" She had heard the story of our celebration when their flight had finally lifted off the ground in Minsk.

"Piña coladas?" Mike feigned shock. "I'll have to check your ID, young lady. I could swear you were just thirteen," he teased.

"Okay, I show you ID," she bantered.

Still wearing his baseball cap, Mike blended pineapple juice, coconut rum, and ice. His face glowed with delight.

Next, he whipped up fancy non-alcoholic drinks for Nikita and Liya. Maria carried the pizza to the table while Vika called the kids in from playing outdoors.

"*Niet!*" sassed Nikita. Just two months shy of his third birthday, he had been steering the police car down the slope of our driveway and crashing into the garage door, over and over. Now, still seated in the vehicle, he backed the rig up the hill with his feet while his mother stood waiting on the porch. As she watched, he lifted his feet and sped downhill.

"*Seychas!*" she yelled after he banged into the door. *Now.* It was The Boss voice I'd heard her use as a child to make Maria toe the line.

Liya, seven going on seventeen, pulled Nikita out from behind the wheel and steered him into the house as he bawled. Long, heartbreaking sobs pulled every stitch of air out of his chest. When he opened his eyes to take a breath, *Dedushka* Mike—Grandpa Mike—handed him and Liya each a kiddie colada. Their eyes grew wide with excitement and Nikita's tears dried up instantly.

After everyone took a seat at the table we lifted our glasses and clinked them together. "I can't believe I drink piña coladas with Gail and Mike!" Vika remarked.

"I can't either!" I agreed. Mike and I exchanged a glance, acknowledging our arrival at the threshold of adult relationships with the twins. They were old enough to consume alcohol *and* they were parenting the children at the table. "Let's take a selfie!" I wanted to commemorate our new family constellation.

After we all leaned in to capture the moment, Nikita tried to grab a slice of pizza before Maria finished cutting wedges.

"*Niet*, Nikita!" Vika scolded.

Scowling, Nikita leaned back in his chair, his eyeglasses skewed. When Maria slipped a crusty slice onto his plate, he dove into it with gusto, smearing his face with ketchup.

"Mmmmmmm," Liya moaned when Maria dropped a wedge on her plate. The kids' eagerness suggested this meal was a favorite.

"Gail?" Maria offered me a slice from the spatula aimed my way.

"Yes, please!" With my first bite, I tasted Belarus— savory, simple, and infused with love.

"You like?" Maria asked.

"Is good!"

"Now, Michael, instead of no *marozhina* if I don't eat my green beans, no alcohol!" Maria teased. Desperate to get her to eat vegetables as a child, Mike had often bribed her with ice cream.

"No alcohol *and* no *marozhina*," he quipped.

Melt-in-your-mouth good and filling, like buttered popcorn, the zucchini zipped around the table as we talked. I turned to Liya.

"It must be difficult for you to be in unfamiliar surroundings where you don't understand the language," I said. Vika translated.

"How can anything be hard, being in this family?" Liya replied. Her declaration of kinship lit my face with a smile. Despite all the ways in which we could never understand each other completely, the bonds holding us together felt tangible, solid, and deep.

CHAPTER 36

❖ Women's Voices

Like characters dancing off the pages of a well-loved book, Vika and Maria waltzed in to meet my writing group. After hearing about the girls for years through stories I'd written, my writer friends could hardly believe they were actually seeing them face-to-face. But, in 2014, they were not the little girls these women knew from the page.

Maria seated herself to my right and gracefully arranged her long legs to one side with her ankles crossed. Vika, sitting straight and tall to my left, settled in with a deep breath. Teabags steeped, perfuming our circle with scents of cinnamon, citrus, and cloves.

"What do you like to do in Belarus when you aren't working?" asked Laura. I was pleasantly surprised when Maria, the less verbal of the twins when they were children, jumped at the opportunity to engage.

"I rest, go with friends, and I drink vodka like man!" Maria replied. I burst into laughter with everyone else, but I wasn't laughing on the inside. Her unexpected response unsettled me. *I hope she's joking.* Despite my protective reflex, I was glad her spunk and independent spirit had remained intact.

We turned to Vika for her response. She was in the final months of a three-year maternity leave from her job, receiving a small stipend, as is customary after giving birth in Belarus. Motherhood and marriage seemed to have made her more reserved than her younger self, yet she was still fully present and engaged.

"I take care with my son, and I play volleyball. My team very good."

"How is your little boy adjusting to being in a foreign country?" Phyllis asked.

"Nikita only two and a half. I worry he be very afraid when we come to America, not leave my side, maybe," Vika began. "On plane he sleep. When he open eyes he look at me and say, 'I love Mike.' They best friends already!" She beamed.

"Sounds like Mike is more of a grandfather than a stranger to your son because you tell stories about him," said Laura. Her comment carried me back to the long-ago day when, sitting with ten-year-old Vika on a mountaintop, I had hoped she would one day share the stories of her trips to America with her own children. I realized, now, that day had come. The memories she had shared with her son had instilled in him the feeling of a safe and loving familial relationship with Mike before they'd ever met. My heart soared as that sank in. And it would soar again later when Vika told me that Nikita had called out for me in the night after they had returned to Belarus.

Ann asked the girls, "What's it like for you, seeing the United States for the first time as adults?"

"In Belarus we don't speak with people we not know, the way you do," Maria answered. "I see Gail and Mike talk with people in stores and bank, for example. Is very interesting to me." Her warmth and openness had fully flowered.

"Maybe not talking to strangers in Belarus dates back to the code of silence practiced during the Soviet era," Laura suggested.

"No," Maria responded. "I think in Belarus many people have difficult life. They not happy and don't want you to be happy." Her response made me wonder if we knew more about the dark side of Soviet history than she did.

Now, as we sipped tea, a sweet intimacy was taking hold between the twins and my friends. At the risk of embarrassing the girls, I asked if they would sing.

"Just one song before it's time for us to leave?"

To our delight, the girls locked eyes and melted into song. Their voices intertwined as if they were a solitary instrument with many strings perfectly tuned, its pure, melancholy voice crying, searching, hoping. That earthy, rich, raw elixir flowed over my skin, rushed into my heart, and pulsed through my veins. In the faces of my friends I saw the glow of enchantment. Tears gathered in my eyes. Each note pulled me deeper. The room where we were sitting, a room I knew well, suddenly became a holy place filled with the resonance of all the loneliness and love and terrible beauty and hope that ever was. Though the lyrics were a mystery to me, the emotion was unmistakable. My heart swelled and ached with unbearable longing and each note left me craving more.

Maria and Vika's song poured light and sorrow into me and into every corner, every crevice of the room. I closed my eyes. *This is the song of the Divine.*

CHAPTER 37

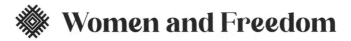 # Women and Freedom

M aria's spirit tanked when she learned, through a friend,
that her Belarusian boyfriend had betrayed her. She
immediately ended the relationship by email. Too distressed
to eat for several days, she stayed home even when we took
the kids out for *marozhina*. Her cheeks caved. The spark in
her eyes blew out. She left the house only to smoke cigarettes,
"to calm my nerves."

"Please, no tell Mike I smoke," she pleaded.

Maria's mood showed no improvement until Ella's
daughter, Anna, offered to take the twins to a Russian
nightclub to dance. Vika jumped at the opportunity. Maria
decided she might as well go too. They stayed out late that
night. When I saw Maria the next morning, her condition
had radically improved. She gleefully informed me she had
met a handsome Russian man and planned to see him again.

"Tonight, Dima pick me up nine o'clock."

My anxiety launched like a rocket. "You don't know
anything about him!" I blurted. Going to clubs with Vika
and Anna had seemed reasonable to me. But going out alone
with a perfect stranger in a foreign country was a different
matter entirely.

"I twenty-five, Gail. Don't worry. He very nice man," she tried to reassure me. But my mama-bear self refused to back down. Too many women in our culture were victims of date rape, or worse.

"You're old enough to make your own decisions in Belarus," I agreed. "But this isn't Belarus. It's different here. You don't know this culture. How would you even get home by yourself if you needed to?" I looked at Mike, pleading with my eyes for him to back me up.

"Take my cell phone with you," he suggested. I glared at him as if he were a traitor.

"I take. If you call, I answer," Maria promised.

"And tell him we'd like him to come in to meet us when he comes to pick you up," Mike added.

"Okay, Michael. I say to Dima my American father like to meet him." Her response struck me as old-world and sweet, but I didn't know how that would keep her safe.

"We need that man's license plate number!" I spewed to Mike when Maria was out of earshot. "You walk outside with them when they leave. Act casual. Wait until they drive away to write it down."

It was almost ten when Maria's date arrived. A bit late, in my opinion, for a first date. Did this tall, muscular fellow with dark blonde hair buzzed close to the scalp hope this would be a booty call? His handshake was firm, and he seemed comfortable with direct eye contact. Did that indicate he was a mature and confident man, or a sociopath? He appeared older than Maria, maybe by five years. Was that a good sign or bad? I couldn't decide. I didn't invite him to sit at that hour, so we all stood awkwardly by the door after Maria made the introductions. I smiled and remained silent while Mike began questioning him.

"Do you live nearby?"

"Not too far. West Seattle." His patient, respectful demeanor seemed to indicate he'd been expecting the third degree and didn't mind. Standing next to him, Maria grinned, enjoying the show.

"Lived here long?" Mike asked next. I had hoped he would first pinpoint *where* in West Seattle this guy lived. But no.

"Yes, twelve years."

"You work in Seattle?"

"Yes, I . . ." Before he could say where he worked, Maria interrupted.

"Okay, Michael? We go now?"

"Yeah, sure. Be safe." Mike waved his hand toward the door.

"Have a good time!" I said, hoping it wouldn't be too good.

As soon as they were outside, Mike hot-footed it into the kitchen, grabbed a bag partly filled with garbage, and rushed it outside as if it were on fire. By the time he reached the trash can, he had burned the license plate number into his memory bank.

After Mike and I turned in for the night, my mind continued to race. As I lay awake, I recalled a story Maria had told me about a Belarusian friend who met her Turkish husband through the internet.

"He Muslim man with two wives, but wives not live together," she had explained. "My friend has own house in Turkey, many nice clothes. Husband come to visit. Is good life, only she can't take her baby to visit family in Belarus."

In my view, polygamous relationships were not equal partnerships. Though I had never met or conversed with a woman married to a man with more than one wife, I assumed that most, if not all of them, were denied the freedom to express their own views and make their own decisions. I believed those freedoms were their birthright, whether they chose to exercise them or not. I couldn't understand how

Maria, a feisty female who drank vodka "like a man," could consider this a good option for her friend. Her positive view of this woman's choice had surprised and troubled me.

"But, what about her freedom?" The emotion in my voice revealed a judgment I had hoped to conceal.

"Maybe for her is good life, Gail. If no one help her in Belarus, maybe she die in street."

Now, as I twisted and turned in bed, waiting for Maria to return from her date, I pondered my Western view of freedom and ruminated on the injustices forcing countless women, even in the United States, into compromised lives in order to survive. That chilling reality kept my mind spinning until three in the morning, when I woke Mike.

"It's three in the morning and Maria isn't back yet!"

"If you're worried, call her." His voice was groggy from sleep.

As promised, Maria answered. "Everything okay, Gail. We outside, talking in car. In ten minutes, I come in house."

First, relief washed over me, then a fantasy arose. *Maybe Maria will marry Dima and immigrate to Seattle!* I drifted off to sleep with my lips curled into a smile.

In the morning, Maria joined me in the kitchen. "Michael is very good husband, Gail," she said with a sarcastic tone and sly smile. "He take garbage out at ten o'clock at night," she teased.

"Oh! You saw him?" I felt like a kid caught with her hand in the cookie jar.

"Yes, I see him. Dima say, 'Mike getting license plate number. Is good papa!'"

"How was your date?"

"He very nice, but we in two countries. We agree we just friends only."

My picture of Maria living in Seattle instantly vanished, leaving me with pangs of disappointment.

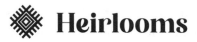 **Heirlooms**

One evening after dinner, Vika popped an unexpected question.

"Gail, you have pictures when you and Mike young? Maria and I like to see."

The twins' desire to know us on another level touched me deeply. It felt like they were opening a door to the kind of intimacy I yearned for.

"Yes! *Odin minute!*" I responded. *One minute.* While I headed off to gather photos, Mike cleared the table, and Liya and Nikita played in the living room.

"Here's a picture of Mike when he was twenty-six, just a year older than you are," I said, returning to the table. The girls howled with surprise when I held up a large photo of a skinny, bare-chested young man with wavy blonde hair down to his shoulders, sitting cross-legged on a rock, amber-tinted aviator sunglasses covering his eyes.

"This *Mike*?" Vika screeched, her voice a full octave higher than normal.

"Yup! I call this 'Buddha Mike'! This was taken in 1976—before I knew him—when he and his friends rode their bicycles all the way across the United States for the Bikecentennial."

"What this, Bikecentennial?" Vika asked.

"Part of the celebration of the two hundredth birthday of the United States. He was a hippie, back in the day. You know what a hippie is?"

"Yes, we know," Maria assured me, laughing. Years later she would explain that, to her, hippies were "interesting people who are different from others, with their own style and their own goals, who listen to their music and constantly enjoy life. If you meet such a person, it is impossible to replace him."

"Here is a picture of me when I graduated from college," I said, handing Vika a photograph of me standing, hands on my hips, in front of the old, weathered barn my parents still owned at that time. A tight sweater, tall boots, and a long, bohemian, brown-and-gold velvet patchwork skirt, made by my sister, accentuated my then-shapely figure. My naturally curly hair was teased into a frizzy aura that completed my unconventional style.

"Your hair!" Vika remarked.

"Yeah, my hair was pretty wild in those days."

"I keep this photograph?" Maria asked.

"Sure!" I said, flattered. "And this is our wedding picture." I handed over a photo of Mike and me with the Unity Church minister who married us on a hill overlooking the ocean in Carmel-by-the-Sea, California. The photo had been taken at our request by a stranger who happened to walk by with her dog just as we finished taking our vows. We hadn't eloped. Our families and friends knew we were in Carmel to be married.

The girls studied the picture of me wearing a peach-colored dress and Mike dressed in a dark blue suit with a peach-colored shirt and tie.

"We had our hearts set on a West Coast wedding, but it would have been complicated for our families to attend," I explained. "So, Mike and I planned a simple ceremony, just the two of us, in a beautiful setting."

I wondered what the girls thought of our nontraditional wedding with no family, no veil, no reception. On the snowy day when Vika had married Fedor, she looked like a winter princess in layers of white lace and chiffon, a sparkling tiara, and a white fur bolero hugging her shoulders. There was music and dancing with friends and family, vodka toasts until early morning, and a limousine excursion through a snow-covered forest, all captured on video. When I watched the video, I couldn't have felt more happy or proud, unless I'd been there seated next to Zoya.

When it came to weddings, Mike and I shared similar values. Our low-key event had suited us and fit our budget. The financial contribution we had made to Vika's wedding had reflected our values, but I would later question whether we had done enough when I realized how much a traditional celebration had meant—in her culture and to her.

"You look so young!" remarked Vika, studying my wedding picture.

"Almost thirty-five! I'll show you my dress," I said, heading to the closet where it hung.

The peach tea-length dress made of soft cotton, with a dropped waist and scalloped cap sleeves and hem, looked more like a garden party dress than a wedding gown. "I bought it at Frederick & Nelson, a special Seattle department store that no longer exists," I said, showing it to the girls.

Suddenly, memories of my mother telling me about her wedding day came floating back. "We were married in a church," she'd told me. "After the ceremony, your grandma and grandpa had a small reception for us at their house. Nothing fancy. We couldn't afford a real honeymoon, so your dad and I stayed in a Detroit hotel for just one night." I tried to imagine them as newlyweds, a nineteen-year-old secretarial school graduate and a twenty-one-year-old farmer.

The fitted dusty-blue jacket Mom wore as a bride eventually found its way to my cedar chest. She also bequeathed to me her beloved Apple Blossom Haviland china, a wedding gift from her brother.

Now, sitting in my kitchen with the twins, I began to see threads of similarity connecting our three wedding stories—Mom's, Vika's, and mine. Themes of limited financial resources and significant absences—my mother's absence at my wedding, and my absence at Vika's wedding.

I began to recognize the deep beauty of our imperfect stories, and to understand those imperfections represented the complexity of authentic relationships, even the shadowy areas. I thought of how my mother's story and heirlooms had strengthened the warp and weft of my world. And I worried this might be my last opportunity to gift Vika and Maria with something of mine they might treasure.

"I'll be right back," I said, stepping out of the room to collect trinkets and treasures from closets and drawers.

Maria was prancing around the kitchen in my wedding dress when I returned. On her tall, slender frame, it looked provincial and frumpy. She curtsied, and we all burst into laughter.

"I guess you won't be wearing my dress for *your* wedding, if you get married!"

I placed the negligee I'd worn on my honeymoon and boxes of mostly costume jewelry on the table. Nikita and Liya came running to join what sounded to them like a party.

"I never wanted diamonds or other precious stones, but there might be something here you'd like to keep," I said.

Liya, now seated at the table with Nikita on her lap, sorted through the jewelry until she discovered a sterling silver charm bracelet and slipped it on her wrist. Holding up her arm, she admired a miniature ice skate dangling among a string of silver charms.

"I received that bracelet as a gift when I was about ten years old," I told her. "Over time I collected all those charms."

"*Krasivaya!*" *Beautiful.*

"Would you like to keep it?"

"Yes, I like!" Her eyes shone.

Vika held up the silky pale-pink nightgown I'd worn on my wedding night. "Ohhh, is very nice," she commented suggestively.

"My friend Nancy bought that for me."

"Verrry good," Maria chimed in.

Vika carefully folded the lingerie and turned her attention to the jewelry. A wide, distinctly vintage band of gold the color of dark honey caught her eye. Smooth on the inside, it featured indentations on the surface that suggested it might have been hand-crafted.

"That was handed down from one of my ancestors, I don't know which one," I explained. "Try it on."

Wearing her own wedding ring on her right hand, as is the custom in her culture, Vika tried the elegant old ring on her left hand. She smiled with satisfaction when it fit comfortably on her middle finger.

"I just remembered something else," I said. From a dresser drawer, I retrieved a sparkling gold ring and handed it to Maria, hoping it would fit her so both girls would go home with a special keepsake.

"Try this," I said. "It's my original wedding band. We bought it in a jewelry store on a trip to San Diego. It's too small for me now." I had replaced it with a sterling silver and gold spinner ring.

Maria tried to slip it on her finger, but it was too small for her too. I frowned with disappointment, but Maria's face lit up.

"I put here," she said, placing one hand on her chest. Then she slipped the ring onto a chain next to a cross she wore around her neck. With that gold symbol of eternity resting next to Maria's heart, the soul of a mother quickened beneath my skin.

That sentimental moment was eclipsed by Nikita when we realized he had dolled himself up with bangles on his arms and strings of pearls around his neck. With a smidge of dried ketchup still clinging to his chin, he looked up grinning.

CHAPTER 39

✦ One Woman's Bridge

Lightning torched the sky over Lake Chelan. Thunder slammed the windows. Jolted awake, Mike and I scrambled down the hall to reassure our flock that we were safe. But Nikita, Liya, and the twins were sleeping, blissfully unaware of the storm.

After I climbed back into bed, I lay awake observing my surroundings through eerie strobes of light. Soon I realized it was I who needed reassurance. The weather didn't frighten me; I was a Midwesterner who enjoyed nature's wild streaks. There was something else. The alarm in me felt nameless.

Each bolt of lightning illuminated the room like the flash of a camera capturing scenes of ordinary life. A bathing suit hanging from the back of a chair. A stack of folded towels resting on a dresser. A baseball cap slung over a door handle. But my senses were distorted. The images I saw appeared strange and surreal, frozen in time. When I closed my eyes, the lightning strikes left me with images that looked like snapshots taken in abandoned houses after the explosion of Chernobyl. Shoes lined up in front of doors. Mixing bowls left behind on countertops. Wedding gowns hanging in closets. Baby cradles. Radios. Letters waiting to be mailed. All contaminated with radiation.

Rain pelted the windows like gunshot. Thunder exploded like bombs. My mind drifted to the updates we'd been hearing about the situation in Ukraine. The United States had just accused Russia of violating a nuclear arms agreement. Russia was building up its forces along the Ukrainian border. Now, unable to sleep, that news gnawed at me. *Would the Belarusian army send troops to support Russia? Would the United States supply Ukraine with weapons that would put Maria and Vika's family members at risk?* I felt sickened.

Don't go there, I told myself. *Enjoy the time you have now*. My instincts told me to immerse myself in the fleeting present, open my heart wide to every precious moment, and quietly bear witness to the dangers.

Exhausted, I wrapped an arm around Mike and, at long last, fell asleep in the wee hours, clinging to my anchor.

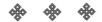

In the morning we awakened to a cool, fresh breeze, the air no longer heavy with the smoky haze of distant wildfires. The mountains stood against the horizon, majestic and clear. All that remained of the storm were puddles on our lanai and tree branches floating in the water. I was thankful my night fears had receded to their daylight place, where I could manage them with little effort.

After breakfast, the temperature climbed. Mike and I took the little ones out in a paddleboat while Vika and Maria sunbathed at the pool. Headed across the east side of Lake Chelan to buy snow cones in the little town of Manson, Mike and I peddled in unison. The waterwheel whirled. Jade-green water shimmered like a silk blanket embedded with thousands of tiny mirrors. Cotton ball clouds rolled across a royal-blue sky as if the colors and contours of the panorama were all part of a freshly painted animation.

Floating across that canvas, I was a happy *babushka*. There was no doubt that I held our two little passengers in the heart of a grandmother. I was a weaver of continuity, connecting generations through a narrative of belonging and love. Though rarely a physical presence in their lives, I was the grandmother who was teaching them it was possible to build bridges across chasms of continents, language, politics, and culture—one snow cone, one UNO game, one Russian pizza, one good-night kiss at a time.

Sporting a life vest, a ball cap, and eyeglasses that magnified his blue eyes and feathery eyelashes, Nikita sat back-to-back with Mike. Their bumping elbows echoed the closeness between them that sometimes baffled Maria and Vika.

"Nikita no understand English, but he and Mike communicate. I don't understand," Maria had commented.

I smiled, remembering the first time the eight-year-old twins had visited Seattle. With only a few words of English, a few words of Russian, hand signals, laughter, and a deck of UNO cards, we too had created our own language and formed a bond that now embraced four generations of their family.

Now, sailing toward Manson, I spotted a dark object bobbing in the crystal-etched waves. "There's a branch! Over there!" I pointed. "Let's go get it!" Seven-year-old Liya, a shining star who consumed information like candy, was sitting back-to-back with me.

"*Da!* Yes!" Liya cried in two languages.

As we turned our little boat in that direction, Nikita squinted one eye against the sunlight. His other eye searched for wood. Ordinarily, he was a boy who ping-ponged from one shenanigan to another, from contagious laughter to heartbreaking wailing episodes. A boy who ate hot dogs with his feet defiantly propped up on the table, one who flung himself off the side of a pool like a jet speeding off a runway, wings spread and landing gear folded back behind him. But now he appeared unusually calm and content. He was on an expedition.

We circled the floating tree limb until it gently collided with our plastic rig. Nikita grabbed it. Liya helped him pull it over the side of our vessel.

"Good job!" Mike called out in his captain's voice.

Wearing my baby-blue hat to protect her face from the sun, Liya turned to Mike. Her pink lips broadened into a smile, serene and satisfied. A soft braid of tawny hair curled over her shoulder.

As we tended to our tiny speck of the universe, clearing debris from our beloved lake, I inhaled the sweet scents of coconut sunscreen, negative ions deposited by the late-night storm, and a piece of cheese Nikita had discarded. A familiar peace carried me back to a moment on our first trip to Lake Chelan with Maria and Vika. As the sun burned silver in the late afternoon, we had been leisurely swimming in deep water, headed back to shore. The girls' faces glowed with contentment. Background screeches and laughter faded away as though a noisy radio had been turned off, leaving only the gentle sounds of breath and water. Our pod felt like a complete universe, more than the sum of our parts. Time seemed to stop and boundaries collapsed. I became one with water, sky, and love.

Now, I was having a similar experience. This time, squeezed together in our little red boat, Nikita and Liya and Mike and I morphed into a cocoon with four hearts beating as one, joined in our common mission.

Collecting branches, we zigzagged toward Manson ensconced by big sky, deep water, and acres of golden-colored hillsides embroidered with green vineyards and fruit trees. I felt swaddled in layers of velvet. My insides hummed with the happiness of knowing that Nikita and Liya were now a part of our story stitched into that landscape.

Soon we reached town and the winds changed. Mike held the boat steady while Liya and I climbed out. As I lifted a wiggly Nikita from the boat to the dock, a wave of grief struck me. The kids would soon be going home to Belarus, and our house would be as quiet as an untapped drum. I knew I was a woman who craved time alone to write, meditate, putter, and read. I yearned for one-on-one time with Mike and friends and nature. Part of me was overdue for solitude. But when my need for quiet eased I would want more hearts thrumming in the house. I wished that I could create the right balance. But that wasn't possible, so I scooped up every precious moment, filling my larder with the chaos and beauty of our global family like caviar to nourish me when I felt starved.

As I transferred Nikita to the dock, I felt his wild impatience revving up, his feet running before they touched down. He pulled at his life vest, wanting it off.

"*Niet*, Nikita," I said, seeing dangers I knew he couldn't understand. Reluctantly, he held my hand until we reached land. Though we were safe, my pulse quickened with an awareness of my inability to protect Nikita and Liya beyond our brief moment together. I could not shelter them from war. All I could do was welcome them across our bridge.

I had dreamed of a world with enough human bridges to support nonviolent resolutions to conflict and put an end to wars—with a Peace Department to replace the War Department in Washington, DC. Now I asked myself, *What good can one woman's bridge do?*

There didn't seem to be any way to influence the current state of affairs surrounding the United States, Russia, Belarus, and Ukraine. Yet wasn't there some chance—even one in a billion—that the joints and footings and wings and towers and parapets of our human bridge were a tiny part of a great network of invisible scaffolding holding our nations together in some semblance of order? I clung to a belief that every intention, every thought, every word, every decision, and every act contains the potential to shape the future and kindle reverence for Earth and all of her inhabitants. And though it might take decades—or even millennia—to manifest a visible tipping point, I was grateful that our bridge was strong and had withstood the test of time for a new generation.

As we ambled into town, Nikita turned to me and raised his arms. His shining eyes filled me with warmth. I leaned down, straightened his lopsided eyeglasses, and picked him up, his soft skin sticky with sweat.

"Gail, *marozhina?*" he asked.

"*Da.* Snow cone!" I replied.

Nikita threw his head back and yipped with glee. Liya punched the air above her head and squealed, "Yessss!"

✸ Epilogue

2023

Our family tree remains strong but battered by separation, war, and the cycle of life. Before the travel restrictions imposed by the COVID pandemic and the rise of the New Cold War, I made a second trip to Belarus, to welcome two new members of the family into the world. Vika had given birth to her second child, a daughter, and Maria had given birth to a son. Although I didn't realize it at the time, it was also a goodbye, the last time I would see Ivan and imbibe the salubrious, soul-stirring music he played on his accordion. Just after his sixtieth birthday, his heart gave out. Grieving the loss of her son, Babushka died six weeks later, brokenhearted. Just weeks after the deaths of those cherished elders, nearly every border in the world was closed in response to the pandemic. By the time those borders began to reopen, Ukraine was a war zone. Travel between the US and Belarus remains off-limits. Sanctions and border closings in Belarus make it almost impossible for the twins to apply for US travel visas. Video calls are our lifeline for staying connected and current on the safety of our loved ones. Fortunately, as of now, they are all safe.

Has our bridge helped to heal our fractured world? I am certain our beautiful silk road benefits the many lives it touches directly and indirectly. I've witnessed the growth and expansion of its reach. And I believe in the ripple effect of healing energy creating a shift in the world's collective unconscious.

Even in the face of unspeakable violence, how could I *not* believe in a benevolent and mysterious force, one that conjured a vision in my childhood and then steered me toward the fulfillment of that forgotten dream, forty years later, against the odds? How could I not believe in portals of transformation after my dream was sparked to life by the confluence of infertility and a nuclear explosion? With enough people willing to play a role, we can create a more empathic world with fewer walls, a world attuned to curiosity and care instead of fear and violence. Each day presents all of us with opportunities to bridge divides in our own communities by acknowledging our shared humanity with gestures of kindness. Eye contact alone can have curative effects.

I dream of one day sitting around a table with my Belarusian family again, elbow to elbow. For now, I am grateful for every visit on my video screen, though the possibility that our calls are under surveillance restricts our conversations. Liya, now an English-speaking teenager with blue-tinted hair hanging over one eye, talks about school, dreams for her future, and highlights of her social life. Maria shares the ups and downs of her busy life as a working mother and helping Zoya at the dacha. Vika sends videos of her daughter dancing and her son playing soccer. Sergey, Elina, the children, and I communicate with waves, smiles, "*Privet*," and "How are you?"

In my bones I know, the bonds that define our constellation will hold even if our last line of communication goes dark. I've learned that relationships bound by the heart can survive grievous obstacles in a splintered world.

❖ Acknowledgments

M ichael McCormick, you are my rock and soul mate. Thank you from the depths of my heart for walking beside me on the holy spiral of life and manifesting this dream with me.

Blessings to all of my friends and family who have accompanied me on the path from heartbreak to Chernobyl and beyond. Though I can't name all of you here, please know that you are deeply appreciated and loved for your support and presence in my life. I couldn't have made this soul-satisfying journey without you.

To the Petrovy family: You have enriched my life beyond measure. Vika and Maria, you are the stars of this story. Thank you for redirecting the arc of my life with your spirit and magic; I admire the strong, beautiful women you are today, *and* you will always be my beautiful swimming fish girls. Zoya, I will be forever grateful that you and Ivan reached across the cultural divide to weave Mike and me into your hearts, your home, and your family.

I'm deeply grateful to Ann Holmes Redding and Laura Bowers Foreman, two extraordinary story doulas, for

introducing me to and guiding me in the process of writing creative nonfiction, encouraging me to write from the
heart of my spiritual truths, and expanding my awareness
of social justice issues, the blindness of privilege, and the
importance of bringing that awareness to my writing. This
book wouldn't exist without your generous dedication,
wisdom, and compassion.

To my beloved past and present writing sisters Kathy
McLean, Floren Lee Sempel, Kathy Grainger, Angeline
Thomas, and the late Phyllis Franklin: I am grateful for
your insight, honesty, encouragement, and willingness to
read umpteen revisions. Your friendship, wisdom, support,
and humor mean the world to me.

Alex and Ella Golovko, without you I might never have
crossed the bridge. Thank you for taking me to your motherland, for your support during the twins' Seattle visits, and all
the joys of our cross-cultural friendship of twenty-five years.

Gratitude to the moon and back to: my dear friend
Jennifer Kropack, who curled up on couches again and again
to read and discuss new chapters and multiple revisions,
from the get-go to the finish line; Nancy Ashley, for the
support you've given me for half a century now, including
proofreading, encouragement, and respites from parenting
during the twins' visits; Nicolette Rose, for your artistic eye,
generosity, and guaranteed laughter; and Linda Post, for
many miles of nature walks and talks that supported me in
managing the emotional roller coaster of writing a memoir.

Heartfelt thanks to the Astrouskaya sisters, Tatsiana and
Olya, for translation and so much more.

Blessings to Nadya Neal and all humanitarians making
the world a better place, including the doctors, dentists, oral
surgeons, beauticians, and others who donated their services
to Children of Chernobyl participants.

Thank you to: Ruth Neuwald-Falcon, in you I found friendship and a copyeditor who puts heart and soul into her work. Sofiia Fedzhora, University of Washington Fulbright teaching assistant, Slavic Languages & Literature, for your help with transliterations and cultural clarity. Michelle Swinea, for your sensitivity reading and enlightening cultural competence analysis. And a shout-out to the We Love Memoirs Facebook group authors (www.facebook. com/groups/welovememoirs/) for so generously sharing your knowledge and support.

Thank you to Brooke Warner, Lauren Wise, and the She Writes Press team for creating a pathway to launch my memoir into the world. I am grateful to be a part of the SWP community of women writers.

Spacibo to all who read *Zoya's Gift. Thank you.* If you enjoyed my story, please let me and others know with a brief review on sites where readers go to find book recommendations.

✤ About the Author

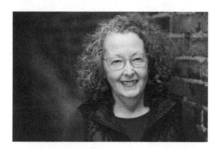

GAIL McCORMICK is a Seattle author and psychotherapist with Midwest roots. She was a finalist in the 2022 Pacific Northwest Writers unpublished memoir competition and took first place for intercultural essays in the 2021 Soul-Making Keats Literary Competition. Her stories have also appeared in the *Timberline Review* and the *Santa Fe Literary Review*. She is the author of *Living with Multiple Chemical Sensitivity: Narratives of Coping*, a nonfiction book in which she addresses the emotional and social impact of living with this environmental illness. She is a former newspaper reporter and biographer with an MS in Community Counseling and a BA in Journalism. She volunteers her services to nonprofit organizations serving immigrants and others affected by dislocation and trauma. Her passions include nature, travel, interfaith spirituality, farmers' markets, and all things organic. She lives with her husband in Seattle.

Visit Gailmccormick.com for book club questions, to schedule an author appearance at your book club meeting, and additional information.

Author photo © Garrett Hanson/Happy Hour Headshot

SELECTED TITLES FROM SHE WRITES PRESS

These Walls Between Us: Lessons from a Friendship Across Race and Class by Wendy C. Sanford. $16.95, 978-1-64742-167-0. In *These Walls Between Us* established feminist author Wendy Sanford, who is white, reflects on her complex lifelong friendship with Mary Norman, who is Black—her formation in a narrow world of class and race privilege, lifting up the writings and social movements that changed her views and her life, and examining a sixty-year interracial friendship that evolved in the context of white supremacy.

On the Ledge: A Memoir by Amy Turner. $17.95, 978-1-64742-225-7. After Amy Turner is mowed down by a pickup truck, she struggles to heal the trauma of her own brush with death—a process that, unexpectedly and despite her resistance, forces her to confront a childhood trauma she thought she resolved long ago: the morning her father climbed out of his fourteenth-floor hotel window and threatened to jump, an event that made national news.

The Odyssey and Dr. Novak: A Memoir by Ann C. Colley. $16.95, 978-1-63152-343-4. Recalling personal experiences of living in Warsaw and Kiev, Ann C. Colley creates a complex, composite portrait of Poland and Ukraine at a time between the fall of the Soviet Union and the recent resurgence of a Russian threat.

Our Song: A Memoir of Love and Race by Lynda Smith Hoggan. $17.95, 978-1-64742-389-6. In 1972 rural Pennsylvania, Lynda and TJ's connection was a magical, interracial, and controversial young love that grew through sharing late-night letters and songs—until their own insecurities let the people around them tear them apart. Four decades later, fate brings them back together—but is it too late?